A E... g 2

D0806723

Feminist Perspectives on The Past and Present
Advisory Editorial Board

AIDS: Setting a Feminist Agenda

Edited by
Lesley Doyal, Jennie Naidoo and Tamsin Wilton

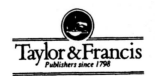

Taylor & Francis
Publishers since 1798

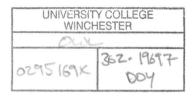
First published 1994
By Taylor & Francis, 11
New Fetter Lane, London EC4P 4EE

Transferred to Digital Printing 2004

Library Catalogue Record for this book is available from the British Library

ISBN 0 7484 0162 8
ISBN 0 7484 0163 6

Library of Congress Cataloging-in-Publication Data are available on request

Series cover design by Amanda Barragry, additional artwork by Hybert ● Design & Type.

Typeset in 11/13pt Times
by RGM Associates, Lord Street, Southport

For all women fighting AIDS.

Contents

Acknowledgments   ix

Introduction   Silences, Absences and Fragmentation   1
                Tamsin Wilton

Section I   **HIV/AIDS and Women**

Chapter 1   HIV and AIDS: Putting Women on the   11
                Global Agenda
                Lesley Doyal
Chapter 2   Women and HIV/AIDS: Medical Issues   30
                Judy Bury
Chapter 3   AIDS: Issues for Feminism in the UK   42
                Diane Richardson

Section II   **The Disputed Body**

Chapter 4   Desire, Risk and Control: The Body as a Site of   61
                Contestation
                Janet Holland, Caroline Ramazanoglu, Sue Scott
                and Rachel Thomson
Chapter 5   Feminism and the Erotics of Health Promotion   80
                Tamsin Wilton
Chapter 6   Visible and Invisible Women in AIDS Discourses   95
                Jenny Kitzinger

Section III   **Masculinities/Femininities**

Chapter 7   Women Have Feelings Too: The Mental Health   113
                Needs of Women Living with HIV Infection
                Sally Dowling

Contents

Chapter 8   Achieving Masculine Sexuality: Young Men's   122
               Strategies for Managing Vulnerability
               Janet Holland, Caroline Ramazanoglu,
               Sue Sharpe and Rachel Thomson

Section IV   Live Issues for a Feminist Agenda

Chapter 9   Feminists, Prostitutes and HIV   151
               Kate Butcher
Chapter 10   Inclusions and Exclusions: Lesbians, HIV and   159
               AIDS
               Diane Richardson
Chapter 11   Against All Odds: HIV and Safer Sex   171
               Education for Women with Learning Difficulties
               Michelle McCarthy
Chapter 12   Time for a Makeover? Women and Drugs in the   183
               Context of AIDS
               Sheila Henderson

Some Useful Organizations in Britain   197
Notes on Contributors   200
Index   203

Acknowledgments

Writing this book has been a long struggle: much longer and much more of a struggle than we anticipated at the start. We would like to thank all our contributors, whose forbearance with delays and rewrites has been exemplary and whose professionalism has been impressive. We would also like to thank Jacinta Evans for being so receptive to the idea in the first place, and Comfort Jegede for whose patience we are grateful. Perhaps the most surprising thing is that the three of us are still good friends!

Silences, Absences and Fragmentation

Tamsin Wilton

When the lengthy process of compiling this book began, little had been written in Britain about women and HIV. While women's issues relating to HIV/AIDS continue to be marginalized, there has recently been a noticeable upsurge of interest accompanied by a flurry of publications. Hence the reader might be forgiven for asking why we need another book on the topic. The simple answer is that this is not a book 'about' women and HIV so much as an attempt to make links between feminism — both as a body of theory and as an activist politics — and the impact on women of the epidemic of HIV infection in Britain. One implication of a feminist as opposed to what might be called a woman-centred approach is that writing about men and masculinity is included here, as part of a critique of the part played by social constructions of gender in this health crisis.

Much has already been achieved, both globally and in the UK, by and on behalf of women living with HIV or its consequences. Specialist HIV/AIDS organizations concerned with women have been established around the world, from the United States to the Netherlands, from England to New Zealand. The Society for Women and AIDS in Africa has projects in many African countries, and many women's health projects in the industrialized and underdeveloped nations alike have established HIV/AIDS programmes, as have a number of family planning organizations (Berer with Ray, 1993). Gay rights groups were often the first to set up HIV/AIDS education and support initiatives, and many of these too are making provision for women, as are specialist AIDS service organizations whether statutory or voluntary. There are Positively Women groups (for HIV-positive women) in major European, Australasian and North American cities, as well as many groups serving minority women living with HIV. The International Community of Women Living with HIV/AIDS set up in July 1992 and based in London, aims to establish a global network of women with HIV, while informal networking, such as that involving women sex workers around the world, has been happening since the early years of the epidemic.

Yet alongside this activity there continue to be too many silences, too much fragmentation of women's limited energies and too great a distance between theory and action. While researchers and activists alike grow increasingly concerned about the possible long-term effects of HIV, there is still an extraordinary failure on the part of those in power in Britain to come to terms with the potential implications of this epidemic. In May 1993 the health minister, Virginia Bottomley, implied that the long-predicted 'heterosexual epidemic' was not happening, and funding for the major AIDS service organizations was cut (Watney, 1993). Yet AIDS is now the major cause of death for women of childbearing age in many cities in Europe and North America. According to the World Health Organization, unprotected heterosexual sex accounts for 70 to 75 per cent of all transmission of HIV worldwide, and an estimated 12 million adults (over 6 million men and 5 million women) — 1 in 250 of the entire world population — are infected with HIV (Panos Institute, 1992). Yet the British government — against the advice of some of its own experts — appears to believe that 'British AIDS' is somehow quite distinct from the pandemic in the rest of the world. This stubborn insularity is likely to have disastrous consequences, particularly for women, who have not yet established the extensive network of support and services which has developed as a central part of the gay community's response to HIV/AIDS.

Activism in the area of health has been one of the most important strands of feminist intervention since the late 1960s. Indeed it is striking that, in the early days of the epidemic, gay men learnt for themselves the painful lessons which the women's health movement had been speaking and writing about for years. The ideological agenda of Western scientific medicine, the hierarchical nature of the medical profession and the powerlessness of marginalized social groups in relation to the medical industry were all put onto the agenda in new ways. Gay men, obliged by the circumstantial pressures of the epidemic to present *as* gay to the medical establishment, ran up against the prejudice, neglect and ignorance so familiar to anyone working in the women's health movement. This did not, of course, mean that women's needs in relation to HIV/AIDS met with different or better treatment from the medical industry than their other health needs. Rather, male homosexuality rapidly became integrated into the disease model for HIV and AIDS, with the result that women were largely ignored.

It is not just the prejudices of Western scientific medicine which gives rise to sensations of *déjà vu*. As with every other major health problem, HIV/AIDS is being dealt with in Britain and around the world by the largely invisible expertise and energies of women carers. As with many other major health problems, women perceive a threat to their autonomy as their reproductive activities are regulated in an attempt to control the global epidemic. At the same time, the power dynamics of heterosexuality make it difficult or impossible for women to protect themselves from HIV, as it has prevented them from avoiding other health hazards in the past. HIV/AIDS is not, then, entirely new and unfamiliar territory for feminism. Yet the links between feminist analysis and HIV/AIDS activism have been frustratingly absent from the agenda of both feminism and AIDS activism in Britain.

The aim of this collection, then, is to make what seem to be essential links between feminism and HIV/AIDS work. To find out how this might be done we have approached a more diverse range of writers than would usually be found in a single collection. It seemed important to ask feminist scholars as well as women engaged more directly in AIDS work, health promoters and educators as well as doctors, women working in long-established feminist arenas whose work was just starting to be affected by the implications of HIV/AIDS as well as women whose work in HIV/AIDS was clearly affected by their feminism. Because these links are just beginning to be made in Britain, this collection inevitably reflects the fragmentary nature of a newly developing approach. Many of the women we approached are overworked, struggling constantly to obtain/ maintain funding and resources, working in poor conditions with little or no support, often isolated: some were ill. This in itself speaks volumes for the conditions under which work in women's health still goes on, particularly in the voluntary sector where women make up the greater part of the workforce.

There are conspicuous absences and silences. For example, women who are caring for people living with HIV/AIDS are here only present as mothers. Clearly this does not reflect the wide range of caring relationships whether professional, voluntary or familial which women are engaged in. Although such absences are perhaps inevitable — a book which sets out to set an agenda can hardly expect to be definitive and all-embracing — they are a clear indication that much still remains to be said and written. Hopefully this collection will encourage further debate among feminists and AIDS activists about the important issues faced by women in this pandemic, about the contribution which feminist theory and practice has to make to the fight against HIV and about the ways in which constructions of gender (together with constructions of race and sexuality) have given this fragile virus such an easy route into the lives of so many millions of people.

As is shown in this book, unequal relations of power between women and men are not simply of academic interest. In the context of HIV/AIDS they are literally life or death issues, for men as well as for women. The women's health movement has much to offer in the struggle to control AIDS, and, in many countries around the world, women's health groups have developed important HIV/AIDS initiatives. Yet in Britain, feminist involvement in AIDS is only beginning, and a number of groups concerned with women's health have so far shown little interest or involvement. Similarly, the extraordinary mushrooming of AIDS service organizations in the voluntary sector has come late to the realization that particular services are needed for women, while AIDS political activism has largely ignored the potentially powerful contribution of feminism. Twelve years into the epidemic the women's movement, still able to call thousands to the streets for pro-choice demonstrations, has been conspicuous by its absence from AIDS activism. The alliances and coalitions necessary to take a stand against the reactionary political AIDS agenda are not happening. This book not only demonstrates that AIDS *is* a feminist issue but also suggests arenas where feminist intervention is long overdue. The authors highlight specifically feminist strategies in support of women living with HIV/AIDS and in the continued fight against the epidemic and its social, political, personal and economic consequences.

In order for activism to be successful, there must be a well-thought-out agenda, and that is what this book aims to outline. The first section explores why HIV/AIDS is an issue not only for women but for feminism. Diane Richardson, in chapter 3, summarizes the strengths and weaknesses of the feminist approach to the epidemic, rejecting many familiar reasons given by feminists for *not* getting involved and illustrating the consequences of a lack of feminist intervention. Her argument that an intervention by women for women is an absolute necessity informs all the other chapters. One of the important challenges to feminism has been the charge that the women's movement has been largely ethnocentric, white and middle-class. Although there are undoubted truths in such criticisms, there has always been a thread of internationalism (which has not always been patronizing or colonialist) running through feminist writing and activism, and nowhere more so than in the women's health movement. Lesley Doyal, whose work has always had a global focus, situates AIDS firmly in the context of the issues facing women outside the relatively privileged confines of the (over) developed West. Sexuality, mothering, prostitution are all aspects of women's lives with crucial relevance to their health, and variations in access to income and wealth mean that they are experienced very differently in the developed and underdeveloped nations.

Clearly the social position of women influences their ability to protect themselves and those close to them from HIV; it is also true that HIV has specific medical implications for women. Judy Bury discusses these in some detail, assessing the risks of transmission during heterosexual and lesbian sex and from mother to baby. She also outlines the clinical manifestations of HIV disease for women and what we know of their distinctiveness from men's experience. From her chapter it becomes clear that the social and the medical intersect in particularly damaging ways for women living with or at risk from HIV.

Feminist theory has identified issues of sexuality as central in women's oppression. This is especially important with respect to HIV/AIDS, where women's ability to practise safer sex is constrained by dominant cultural constructs of 'normal' and acceptable female sexuality. Janet Holland, Caroline Ramazanoglu, Sue Scott and Rachel Thomson have spent many years researching the problems which young British women face in negotiating sexual encounters with their male partners. Their findings have made clear the imbalance of power inherent in such encounters. Siting their enquiry firmly in/on the body, they deal in chapter 4 with the need for heterosexual women to 'come to terms with the ways in which the social construction of masculinity and femininity estranges women from their bodies' (p. 61), and hence the need for HIV/AIDS health promotion to recognize the inappropriateness of demands that women take control in/of heterosex.

But how are such regimes of power instituted and maintained? Partly, at least, by cultural means, by the deployment of representations of sexuality, and it is this which Tamsin Wilton takes as her theme. She suggests that the harm of pornography lies not in its explicitness (indeed, explicitness is, she argues, necessary for safer sex education/promotion) but in its complicity in the construction of female sexuality as passive and male as active. Furthermore, she finds that safe sex promotional materials themselves, using an already established semiotic vocabulary taken from pornography, reinforce precisely those constructions of male and female sexuality which Holland *et al.* have found to be so harmful to young women negotiating sex with male partners.

Jenny Kitzinger comments that AIDS itself has been firmly constructed as a 'male disease' and women as representing a risk to men. This not only influences the provision of services for women but also enables the sexist and oppressive construction of 'women' within and by AIDS discourse. This discourse thereby acquires a covert patriarchal agenda and becomes identified with the larger cultural project of maintaining women's subordination, and so we see the operation of a truly vicious double bind by which women who have sex with men are systematically disempowered.

The third section of the book is concerned with gender, with masculinity and femininity as they operate within institutions and relationships. Sally Dowling, a practising counsellor working with newly diagnosed HIV-positive clients, draws attention to the ways in which the social construction of women as mothers and carers, together with the construction of AIDS as 'masculine', can have grave implications for the mental health needs of HIV-positive women. Very little has been written, either in the feminist or mental health literature, about the emotional experiences of women with HIV infection or HIV disease and this in itself indicates the relatively low priority accorded to women in this field. As Dowling suggests, counselling practice informed by a radical feminist perspective is urgently needed.

Most feminist work has traditionally focused on women and prioritized women's issues. However, there has recently been much debate about the conflict between the need to change men's behaviour on the one hand and, on the other, unwillingness to expend energy on men in what appears to be a traditionally 'feminine' way. In the case of feminist writing about HIV/AIDS, some writers (e.g. Wilton and Aggleton, 1990) have called for a specific focus on masculinity, deploring the invisibility of the heterosexual male 'norm' in AIDS discourse and pointing out that it is precisely *men's* behaviour which puts women at risk. It is exciting to be able to include here Janet Holland, Caroline Ramazanoglu, Sue Sharpe and Rachel Thomson's account of their latest research into young men and masculinity. In chapter 8, they present a detailed picture of the pressures on and the strategies employed by young heterosexual men to claim and proclaim a (fragile) masculinity; strategies and pressures which we must understand and challenge if we are to achieve heterosexual autonomy and safety for women. Their work promises to be not only crucial to the promotion of safer sex but also a rich source of insights into the processes whereby gender-appropriate sexual behaviour is performed and maintained.

Feminism, although offering a crucial perspective on this epidemic, is far from exempt from oppressive and/or exclusionary practices, as several chapters in the final section remind us. Kate Butcher raises some awkward questions about what an appropriate feminist response to prostitution should be, a debate which has a long history within the women's movement and one with particular relevance in the context of HIV disease. Seen as important only insofar as their work poses a risk to their male clients, prostitution of course makes *women* extremely vulnerable to infection, and it is their social and economic marginalization which ensures that for many women there is little alternative. The social factors which structure women's lives again emerge within Butcher's analysis as the starting point for effective HIV/AIDS prevention work.

Another vulnerable and marginalized group, all too often unrecognized by feminist writers, are people with learning difficulties. Only very recently has it been argued that people with learning difficulties have the right to an autonomous sexuality; their lot at the hands of their 'carers' has all too often been repression or exploitation. Michelle McCarthy offers a bleak and painful insight into the sexual lives of women with learning difficulties, arguing that it is only by approaching this issue from an explicitly feminist perspective that we may begin to understand their experiences. She does not allow us the comfortable escape of casting these women into the role of 'other', reminding us that their experiences of abuse or of a sexuality devoid of pleasure were, until recently, the norm for all women.

Lesbians continue to be poorly served by HIV/AIDS health promotion. Inadequate research into women-to-women sexual transmission of HIV, coupled with widespread ignorance concerning lesbian sexual practices, have resulted in conflicting messages about how lesbians may protect themselves from HIV infection. The premature labelling of AIDS as a gay plague resulted in a perceptible increase in hostility towards the gay community by the heterosexual majority, a hostility directed towards lesbians as well as gay men. Some gay men have reacted angrily to lesbians demanding information about safe sex, while some lesbians living with HIV have experienced isolation and suspicion from their communities. Diane Richardson's chapter on lesbians and AIDS is an important and timely contribution to a debate that continues to be largely silenced.

One reason why the response to this epidemic has frequently been so hampered by denial and so ineffective is that it appeared in the early days to affect only the most stigmatized and marginalized groups in the industrialized West, gay men and injecting drug users. Women who inject drugs may be forgiven for thinking that feminism has little to offer them, since feminism has demonstrated little interest in women's recreational drug use or addiction.[1] Yet injecting drug use is, and will continue to be, one of the ways in which women become infected with HIV, and gender is at least as important an issue in drug use as it is in sex. Sheila Henderson's chapter offers a clear outline of the complex issues involved, and places women's injecting drug use firmly where it has long belonged, on the feminist agenda.

Taken together, these diverse pieces present a complex picture of gender, sexuality and the various oppressions which intersect with them to keep women marginalized, silenced and at risk. But because they develop from involvement and activism, the book becomes not a cause for depression but an impetus to action. It is, more than anything else, a catalyst. It suggests theoretical models for understanding and challenging the social factors which are conducive to the spread of HIV among women and among men, as well as offering models of good practice for working with and for women. We hope it will lead to change.

Note

1 Lesbian feminism is the honourable exception to this; much has been written about substance abuse by lesbians and there is a clear theoretical model linking addiction to the need to develop survival strategies in a hostile and homophobic society. See for example essays in Shernoff and Scott (1988).

References

BERER, M. with RAY, S. (1993) *Women and HIV/AIDS: An International Resource Book,* London, Pandora Press.

DOYAL, L. (1993) 'Changing Medicine: Gender and the Politics of Health', in GABE J. and WILLIAMS, P. (eds) *Challenging Medicine,* London, Tavistock.

PANOS INSTITUTE (1992) *The Hidden Cost of AIDS — The Challenge of HIV to Development,* London, Panos Pulications.

SHERNOFF, M. and SCOTT, W. (eds) (1988) *The Sourcebook on Lesbian/Gay Healthcare,* Washington, National Lesbian/Gay Health Foundation.

WATNEY, S. (1993) 'Paying for AIDS', *Gay Times,* May.

WILTON, T. and AGGLETON, P. (1990) 'Young People and Safer Sex', paper given at the First Scandinavian Conference on Safer Sex, Stockholm.

Section I

HIV/AIDS and Women

Chapter 1

HIV and AIDS: Putting Women on the Global Agenda

Lesley Doyal

Introduction

HIV and AIDS are not perceived as significant problems by most women in the United Kingdom (Richardson, 1987; O'Sullivan and Thomson, 1992). Official figures underestimate the real total, but relatively few appear to have been infected with the HIV virus so far and even fewer have developed AIDS. By January 1993 2,370 British women had been identified as HIV-positive compared with 16,640 men, and 466 had been reported as having AIDS compared with 6,463 men (Communicable Disease Report, 1993). HIV and AIDS have remained low on the feminist list of priorities and the specific needs of women have received relatively little attention in the planning of preventive and treatment services.

Closer examination of the global pandemic suggests that gender issues in HIV and AIDS cannot be ignored in this way. While future patterns of HIV/AIDS infection in the UK cannot be predicted with total accuracy, there continues to be an upward trend in the number of cases notified and in the proportion of women among those infected. Across Europe as a whole, 75,000 new cases of HIV infection were notified in 1991, with the rate rising especially fast among women (Mann *et al.*, 1992, p. 33).

In the UK the number of men with AIDS rose by 8 per cent between January 1991 and December 1992 and the number of women by 18 per cent (Communicable Disease Report, 1993). Though these numbers are still small and include infections contracted outside the UK, the risk of further spread remains. Closer scrutiny of the experiences of women in other parts of the world is therefore essential if we are to identify the most effective strategies for containing the spread and for caring for those who are affected whether in Britain or elsewhere in the world.

Is AIDS Becoming a Women's Disease?

The AIDS pandemic is now extremely complex, consisting of a number of smaller and constantly changing epidemics which affect individuals, communities and nations in a multiplicity of different ways. These epidemics themselves reflect variations in the living and working conditions of men and women around the world. It would therefore be inappropriate to envision any future epidemic in the UK on the basis of a comparison with women's experiences in Africa, Asia or the United States. However, the development of the pandemic outside,the UK does offer certain important — and transferable — lessons about the relationship between sex, gender, HIV and AIDS.

Worldwide, heterosexual intercourse is now the most common route for the transmission of the HIV virus (Mann *et al.*, 1992, p. 31). Sex between men remains the most frequent source of infection in the United States and Europe, but here too, the proportion of HIV infections transmitted through heterosex is increasing. Women also form a significant proportion of those infected through intravenous drug use. Hence, both women and children are becoming HIV positive and developing AIDS in ever greater numbers.

By early 1992 best estimates suggested that about 12.9 million people in the world were HIV-positive, of whom 1.1 million were children, 4.7 million women, and 7 million men. Thus about 40 per cent of seropositive adults in the world are female (Mann *et al.*, 1992, p. 29). About one-fifth of these already have AIDS and about 2.5 million have died. The proportion of male: female among those known to be infected by HIV is estimated to be 10:1 in Eastern Europe, 8.5:1 in the US and 2:1 in South-East Asia (Mann *et al.*, 1992, p. 31). In a number of African countries the numbers of men and women who are HIV positive have now equalized, and in some, women are now said to be in the majority (Mann *et al.*, 1992, p. 31; Berer with Ray, 1993, p. 46).

Thus AIDS can no longer be represented as an epidemic among gay men. It is a potentially fatal disease affecting both sexes in huge numbers. If we are to understand the implications of this development, a number of important questions need to be explored. How are women united in their vulnerability to HIV and AIDS and how are they divided by their economic and social circumstances? Can we draw general conclusions about the HIV/AIDS epidemic among women and if so what are their implications for policies in Britain and around the world?

All the Same under the Skin?

Women are united in their biological vulnerability to HIV. It is now clear that they are at greater risk then men of contracting HIV both from an individual act of intercourse and also from each sexual partnership. This 'biological sexism' applies not only to HIV but to most other sexually transmitted diseases (Hatcher *et al.*, 1989). A woman has a 50 per cent chance of acquiring gonorrhoea from an infected male partner while a man has a 25 per cent chance if he has sex with an infected woman. In the case of HIV there is still considerable debate about the precise size of this differential, but it is clear that women are at greater risk.

The reasons for this are complex and derive from the fluid dynamics of unprotected sex, in which the male deposits several millilitres of potentially infectious semen over the surface of his partner's vagina, where it is likely to remain for some time. The risk is further increased by the fact that the virus is more heavily concentrated in semen than in vaginal secretions and by the greater permeability of the mucous membranes of the vagina compared with those of the penis.

Women's greater biological vulnerability to sexually transmitted diseases other than HIV is a problem in its own right but it also increases their risk of contracting HIV itself. Untreated genital infections, especially genital ulcer disease (chancroid), syphilis and genital herpes, all predispose to HIV infection. Women with sexually transmitted diseases tend to remain symptomless for longer than men and untreated lesions give easier access to the virus (Wasserheit and Holmes, 1992; Laga, 1992). In Africa, women's greater biological vulnerability to sexually transmitted diseases in general and AIDS in particular appears to balance out the increased risk men incur through more frequent sexual encounters, resulting in equality between men and women in rates of HIV infection.

Thus all women bring greater biological vulnerability to a potentially dangerous sexual encounter. As we shall see, this is frequently reinforced by cultural, social and economic factors which place major constraints on their ability to protect themselves from infection.

HIV and Patriarchy

Any attempt to analyze the nature of those constraints must begin with the inequality inherent in most heterosexual encounters (Wilkinson and Kitzinger, 1993). One consequence of the current pandemic is that sexual meanings and practices have come under much greater scrutiny than at any other time in human history. While further research is needed, preliminary findings have confirmed many of the more anecdotal accounts of male domination emerging from feminist movements around the world.

Sex between men and women (or between women and women, and men and men) is not always the same. It varies between historical periods and in different societies, between classes and racial groups and between individuals (Foucault, 1978; Weeks, 1986). It is not merely a spontaneous and instinctive biological act but is socially constructed in complex and highly symbolic ways. Yet despite such differences of time and place, both the discourses and the practice of heterosex have certain core elements. Almost everywhere, primacy is accorded to male desire and women are cast as the passive recipients of male passion.

The general acceptance of such beliefs in varying cultural contexts is striking, and provides the setting within which many women have to negotiate greater control in their heterosexual encounters. Many feel they have no right to assert their own needs and desires in a situation where the male partner's wants are seen to be paramount. They feel unable to assert their wish for safe sex, for fidelity, or for no sex at all. These beliefs may not simply kill a woman's desire; they may also lead directly to her contracting HIV.

Sex as a Survival Strategy

This cultural domination of heterosex is reinforced by broader gender inequalities in income and wealth. For many women, their economic security -- sometimes their very survival — is dependent on the support of their male partner. Sexual intercourse done in the way that he desires may well be the price they pay for that support. Hence many women's ability to control their exposure to HIV may be limited by their financial dependence. Requests for safer sex can be made, but if they are ignored most women will have few options, as the Ugandan MP Maria Matembe has described:

> The women tell us they see their husbands with the wives of men who have died of AIDS. And they ask 'What can we do? If we say no more they'll say pack up and go. But if they do where do we go?' They are dependent on the men and they have nowhere to go. What advice can we give these women? (Panos Institute, 1990, p. vi)

This widespread economic dependence on men is not, of course a 'natural' phenomenon. It stems on the one hand from the continuing discrimination many women still experience in the education system and the labour market, and on the other from the social responsibility they acquire for the children they bear.

The links between economic support and heterosex can take very different forms ranging from relationships with no financial implications at all through to commercial sex work where specific acts are performed solely for money. In most societies sex is implicitly assumed to be a husband's right in return for supporting his family. Indeed this continues to be enshrined in most national legislation, with rape being deemed impossible within marriage. In some societies there is a clear dichotomy between marriage and other forms of sexual and economic exchange but in others there is a continuum of different types of sexual services (Seidel, 1993, p. 188).

In parts of Africa for instance, many women have long-term boyfriends on the explicit understanding that they will receive money in return. Indeed there is evidence that a growing number of young girls are making arrangements of this kind as the only means for funding their education (de Bruyn, 1992, p. 255; Bassett and Mhloyi, 1991, p. 150). Whatever the form of sexual/economic exchange, women will be constrained in their attempts to protect themselves — the greater the degree of financial dependence, the greater the constraint.

In many parts of the world, social pressures are now pushing an increasing number of women towards selling sex for subsistence under circumstances that may seriously damage their health. A recent study of black women in mining towns in South Africa revealed that the decision to provide sexual services is usually an economic one:

> Women talk of 'spanning donkeys' (hopana dipkola) or 'spanning oxen' (hopana dikhomo) when describing prostitution. In other words women harness men's desires to work for and support them. Taking sexual partners is a way to supplement meagre salaries or replace them. (Jochelson *et al.*, 1991, p. 167)

As one women described it:

> I worked for six months and saw that it's better to span. I send home money for my children to get something to eat, just think what it's like if you have no place, no money, no husband. (ibid.)

In parts of Asia too, many more women are beginning to sell sex and the rate of spread of HIV among commercial sex workers is extremely rapid. Recent figures indicate that infection is rising rapidly in India's urban slums. In the red light district of Bombay the rate of seroprevalence rose from 0 to 25 per cent between 1986 and 1989 and about 20 per cent of the 100,000 to 300,000 women sex workers are now HIV positive (Panos Institute, 1992, p. 15). Similar increases have been noted among female sex workers in Thailand, where the earning potential of international 'sex tourism' draws many young women in from the countryside. Selling sex is likely to pay as much as twenty-five times more than any other job open to uneducated young women, and many are under considerable pressure to help their families pay off growing debts (Ford and Koetsawang, 1991, p. 409). In the Northern region, around Chiang Mai more than 40 per cent of women working in brothels are already HIV-positive (*ibid,* p. 406).

As well as economic and social insecurity many women also have to face the threat of physical violence. Reports from around the world suggest that many men respond with a beating to women's attempts to protect themselves from HIV infection. Not surprisingly many prefer to risk unsafe sex in the face of more immediate threats to their physical wellbeing. The Ugandan sociologist Mere Kisekka has illustrated the problem with a case from Kampala.

> Recently on the outskirts of the city came a husband who allegedly assaulted his wife because she refused to have sex with him. She was fearful that his former philandering ways might have inflicted him with the disease. For almost two years he totally ignored her until now. But she wanted no part of him. His reaction was to viciously beat her up. Few would condone such behaviour. But then again, as one sympathetic man noted on the incident: 'She was his wife. He had every right to sleep with her if he so wished'. (Kisekka, 1990, p. 40)

For some women, refusal to consent to intercourse may also be the trigger for rape or other sexual abuse (Seidel, 1993, p. 179). Tragically, this may heighten the danger of infection because lacerations or bleeding make it easier for the HIV virus to enter a woman's bloodstream.

Thus women's sexual behaviour is the outcome of a complex set of internal calculations and interpersonal negotiations which cannot be understood outside the context of their cultural, social and economic environment. Not surprisingly it is the poorest women who have the least autonomy, run the most frequent risks and are most likely to be infected. As Bassett and Mhloyi (1991, p. 146) have observed in Zimbabwe, 'For many women faced with divorce or dire poverty on the one hand and the risk of HIV infection on the other, the choice becomes one of "social death" or biological death'.

HIV, AIDS and Poverty

The growing numbers of women with HIV and AIDS are concentrated in the poorest countries — in the 'third world'. At present the majority are in sub-Saharan Africa where the migrant labour system, rapid urbanization and frequent 'low-intensity' wars have combined with growing landlessness and poverty to create an environment which is ripe for the spread of all sexually transmitted diseases and of HIV in particular (Zwi and Cabral, 1991; Jochelson *et al.*, 1991; Bassett and Mhloyi, 1991). Latest estimates suggest that nearly 4 million African women are now HIV positive — 83 per cent of HIV infections among women worldwide (Mann *et al.*, 1992, p. 89). In South-East Asia, current figures are much lower but the rate of increase is extremely rapid, and current estimates suggest that by the year 2000 the largest number of infections will be in Asia and Oceania (*ibid.*, p. 107).

But HIV-positive women are not confined to the poorest parts of the world. In the United States, the richest country of all, some 130,000 women are now thought to be infected with the virus (Mann *et al.*, 1992, p. 83). Again, it is the poor who are most at risk. Black and Latina women are much more likely to be infected than white women, with women of colour accounting for about three-quarters of all women with AIDS in the United States (Banzhaf, 1990, p. 81). Many are intravenous drug users who have little chance of achieving social equality, and sex may be the only commodity they can sell to support themselves and their families (Worth, 1989). For many this means unsafe sex with multiple partners, making the crackhouses of the 1990s as dangerous for women as the bath-houses of the early 1980s were for gay men (Anastos and Marte, 1991, p. 193). Drug use or sex with infected men may be the only means of escape from the impoverishment and marginality of their daily lives. As a counsellor working in inner-city New York put it:

> If the only ways of escape people have are through drugs and sex
> — which offer a rare chance to feel like a complete human being
> — and both of these are closely linked with AIDS then what

hope is there of addressing the issue of AIDS prevention? (Panos Institute, 1990, p. 35)

We have seen that women are biologically more vulnerable than men to HIV infection. In most societies, their own freedom of sexual choice is limited, and many have little control over that of their partners, and this is reflected in their growing visibility in the global AIDS pandemic. Women themselves are seeking ways to transform this situation, but evidence from around the world indicates that most HIV and AIDS prevention programmes have failed to come to terms with their particular needs and circumstances.

Gender Bias in Prevention Programmes

Most HIV prevention programmes attempt to persuade people to change their sexual behaviour — and in the case of women that of their partners too. They assume that men and women can be given knowledge which will lead them to make rational decisions to practise safer sex and then to implement those decisions. However, they often fail to recognize the difficulties facing those women who attempt to do this.

Recent research among Latina women in New York has shown that many are becoming increasingly assertive in their interaction with sexual partners. One Hispanic woman said of her boyfriend: 'Mine doesn't have a choice. Like it or not he has to use a condom with me. Or else nothing can happen. He will suffer for months'. Another black woman reported: 'I insist that he use protection. And if he doesn't want to, then he don't get the goodies. That's all'. (Kline *et al.*, 1992, p. 453). But others feel unable to make such demands, and some men resist all attempts to change them. Women cannot use condoms in the way most government programmes recommend. Instead they must persuade men to do so, and this can be an extremely difficult task (Worth, 1989; Ulin, 1992; Holland *et al.*, 1990; Carovano, 1991).

In one piece of action research in Zaire, sixty married women in a church group attempted to persuade their husbands to use condoms. One-third of the husbands refused without discussion and many of these were angry and hostile, one refusing his wife 'housekeeping' and suggesting she go out and 'hustle'. One-third of the men convinced their wives that there was no risk (perhaps correctly). Only one-third agreed to use the condom (Grundfest Schoepf *et al.*, 1991, p. 199).

Reports from many countries have documented women's fears of family conflict, violence and economic loss if they try to enforce condom use. Young girls in particular often fear that they will be accused of mistrust, of 'not loving him enough', or of being too sexually assertive (Holland *et al.*, 1990). For them, the problem may be not so much economic or social dependence as a fear of challenging dominant ideas about heterosex — of asserting their own needs and putting male pleasure in second place. When Holland and her co-researchers studied the sexual behaviour of teenage girls in the UK, they found that 'The main thing standing between young women and safe sex is the men they are with'. (Holland *et al.*, 1990).

Most prevention strategies also recommend faithfulness within a sexual relationship as a means of ensuring that sex is safe. However, this will mean little to the millions of women who already confine their sexual activity to their husband or long-term partner. It has been estimated that between 50 per cent and 80 per cent of all HIV-infected women in Africa have had no sexual partners other than their husbands (Reid, 1992, p. 659). A recent study in Rwanda found that two-thirds of women claimed to have had only one lifetime partner, but 21 per cent of these women were HIV-positive (Allen *et al.*, 1993, p. 55). Thus the risk for many women comes not from their own sexual behaviour but from that of men over whom they have little control.

This reality goes largely unrecognized as many campaigns continue to treat women as 'moral guardians' giving them responsibility for controlling not only their own behaviour but that of their partners. In Uganda, for instance, government education campaigns have not only exhorted women themselves to adhere to strictly monogamous behaviour — called 'zero grazing' — but also to require their husbands to do the same (Kisekka, 1990).

Of course women as well as men may ignore calls for safer sex. Some reject the 'aesthetics' of sex with a condom or the meanings associated with it. A black woman from New York with an HIV-positive partner reported:

> I don't like them. Because it's some kind of chemical, the stuff it's made from, the stuff they have on those Trojans. And it rubs off into the woman by being rubber, and it causes a lot of problems too. (Kline *et al.*, 1992, p.452)

A Hispanic woman in the same study commented:

> You get embarrassed going to the store. When you go to the store you tell the person at the counter you want a pack of condoms and then he'll shout it where everyone in the store will know what you are there for. (*ibid.*)

A more fundamental obstacle is the fact that most women wish to become mothers at some point in their lives and most will want to have more than one child. Unless male fidelity can be assured, conception cannot be combined with safe sex. This dilemma has been highlighted by Noeleen Kaliba, Director of the AIDS Support Organisation in Uganda, who reported the feelings of one young woman who came to her for counselling. She could not protect herself from HIV, the woman said, because 'Babies and condoms don't go together, non-penetrative sex is no sex at all for a man, and it is a woman's responsibility to bear a child' (Carovano, 1991, p. 135).

Of course many men also wish to become parents and the number of children a man fathers may be seen as an important measure of his potency. But for women the need for children is usually more profound. In many societies motherhood represents the only route to status, identity and personhood, and ultimately to security and support in old age. Indeed, it may be the only way a woman can keep a husband or partner, since in many communities a man is expected to leave a wife who does not 'give' him children. As a result, many women feel forced to choose between motherhood and safe sex — to put their own life at risk in order to bring another one into the world. As one Ugandan woman put it, 'I don't mind dying but to die without a child means that I will have perished without trace. God will have cheated me' (de Bruyn, 1992, p. 255).

Equal Opportunities in Treatment?

If a woman becomes infected, gender inequalities also affect her survival chances and the quality of care she receives. There is evidence from many countries that women's lower social status and greater poverty means that they have less access than men to health care. Research in a number of the poorest countries shows that girls are less likely than boys to receive medical care and this discrimination continues into adult life (WHO, 1992; Ravindran, 1986; Kynch and Sen, 1983; Jacobson, 1992).

In most of the developed countries, sex differences in access to medical care have been eliminated by the development of national health systems. However, the United States remains a notable exception. Many women with low incomes are not able to get care, with women from ethnic minorities being especially neglected (Davis and Rowland, 1991). Along with inadequate living and working conditions, lack of care is an important factor contributing to the high levels of morbidity experienced by women in many parts of the world (WHO, 1992). It also exacerbates the growing damage caused by sexually transmitted diseases in general and HIV/AIDS in particular.

The incidence of sexually transmitted diseases has been rising rapidly in many countries. Among pregnant women in the third world, gonorrhoea rates are now 10–15 times higher, chlamydia rates 2–3 times higher and syphilis rates 10–100 times higher than rates among comparable women in the industrialized countries (Wasserheit and Holmes, 1992, p. 13). This is part of a growing burden of gynaecological problems borne by some of the world's most disadvantaged women (Bang *et al.*, 1989). Sexually transmitted diseases are also a major problem among some groups in the United States with gonorrhoea, syphilis and chancroid increasing at epidemic rates among black and Hispanic women in parts of the inner cities (Aral and Holmes, 1991). Women are the most seriously affected because they often experience no symptoms until the disease is well advanced, and have greater difficulty obtaining care once the problem is recognized. Untreated disease can cause severe complications such as pelvic infection, ectopic pregnancy and infertility as well as facilitating the transmission of HIV and thereby contributing to the growing volume of female deaths from AIDS.

AIDS cannot be cured, but survival after diagnosis, as well as quality of life, are directly affected by the availability of medical services. Though the anti-viral drugs currently available are not proving to be as effective as many had hoped, certain other drugs are valuable in treating opportunistic infections such as *Pneumocystis carinii* pneumonia (PCP), and in providing symptom relief. Yet women often experience great difficulty in gaining access to such care. In the poorest parts of the world, where AIDS is commonest, health care budgets are so small that neither sex can expect sophisticated treatment, but even here resources are spent disproportionately on men. According to a recent survey none of the new care and support programmes either operating or being planned in Uganda, Rwanda, Zambia and Zimbabwe are designed to meet the particular needs of women (Seidel, 1993).

In the United States too, a variety of factors including gender and race have been shown to influence quality of care. This has been highlighted in the debate about access to drug trials. So long as a disease has no known cure, clinical trials of new drugs may represent the only hope for survival. Hence entry to the trials of new AIDS drugs has been keenly sought (Denenberg, 1990a). However, most women have been excluded, usually on the grounds that their numbers are too small to give an adequate sample, or that any potential pregnancy could be endangered and the foetus harmed. Possible damage to a newborn child is clearly a matter for concern, but it is not an insurmountable problem. Entry to trials is now being opened up and this process needs to be continued to give women early access to potentially valuable drugs (Berer with Ray, 1993, p. 31). Even more importantly we need to know about any sex differences in the safety and efficacy of new drugs and this can only be achieved by testing them on a representative sample of patients (Rosser, 1992).

This pattern of male bias in clinical medicine is not confined to HIV and AIDS, as research in other areas has recently documented (Office of Research on Women's Health, 1992). However, the bias is particularly noticeable in the case of HIV and AIDS since in most countries men have historically been the major uses of services. In the United States gay men have been heavily involved in the organization and funding of both research and treatment facilities, and concentration on their needs and priorities was entirely appropriate in the early stages of the epidemic. But as more women become infected, the lack of specific knowledge of both their clinical and their psychosocial needs is posing particular problems, not just in the United States itself but in many other parts of the world, where American research continues to provide the basis for most care and treatment (WHO, 1989b).

We still know very little about sex differences in the transmission, the symptoms and the progression of HIV and AIDS — in its 'natural history' (Denenberg, 1990b). Data derived from the experiences of men cannot simply be extrapolated to women, and a number of important questions remain to be answered. Very little is known about the specifics of HIV transmission to women or its biological consequences, and we need to explore both the social and the biological factors which lead to women becoming infected at a younger age than men (Reid, 1992, p. 664). Another area of particular ignorance is the relationship between HIV/AIDS and pregnancy (Brettle and Leen, 1991, p. 1284).

Existing studies offer contradictory results and despite the fact that a large number of at-risk pregnancies have now taken place, we still know very little about either the influence of pregnancy on the progression of HIV/AIDS or the impact of HIV/AIDS on the outcome of pregnancy. The vertical transmission of the virus between mother and baby is also little understood, though the woman's state of health and the stage of her illness do appear to be significant factors in determining whether or not the child becomes infected. The proportion of children of HIV-positive women who are themselves infected varies between about 15 per cent and 40 per cent, with the children of poor mothers being most at risk (Berer and Ray, 1993, p. 74).

Thus women who contract HIV may face even greater uncertainty than infected men. This often begins with the problems they face in getting a correct diagnosis, since existing diagnostic guidelines pay little attention to symptoms such as thrush, herpes, menstrual problems and cervical cell abnormalities that seem to characterize the early stages of the disease process in many women (Denenberg, 1990b; Marte, 1992; Berer with Ray, 1993, pp. 15–18; Brettle and Leen, 1991). Indeed, a significant number are diagnosed only during pregnancy or when their child is found to be HIV-positive.

At present the combination of unequal or delayed access to care and the male bias in existing knowledge means that women in both rich and poor countries have a shorter life expectancy than men after a diagnosis of AIDS. In Brazil, for instance, the average woman survives only 5–8 months, while a man survives about three times as long (de Bruyn, 1992, p. 250). In New York City a similar gap exists, with man surviving an average of 374 days after diagnosis compared with 298 for women (Rothenberg *et al.*, 1987, p. 1298). The survival rate for black and Hispanic women is shorter than that for white women and women using injection drugs have a particularly poor prognosis.

As well as the clinical differences between men and women, their different psychosocial circumstances may also require a specialized response which male-oriented services are ill-equipped to provide. HIV-positive women who become pregnant, or who consider doing so, have to make major choices and face potentially traumatic emotional experiences. Intrinsically difficult decisions are further hampered by lack of knowledge about the risks involved. The possibility of giving birth to a terminally ill child is daunting, as is the inevitability of one's own death when the child is still small. Yet many decide to go ahead, and one in eighty births in New York City now involve HIV-positive mothers (Faden *et al.*, 1991, p. 309).

Pregnant women affected by HIV or AIDS need positive help with housing, employment and income support as well as health care, but too often they become the objects of negative medical surveillance, receiving fragmented and inappropriate treatment (Walker, 1990). Indeed, some are denied access to any care at all (Berer with Ray, 1993, p. 96). Experience in the United States in particular suggests that many have their right to informed consent jeopardized by pressure to avoid a pregnancy or to have it terminated (Faden *et al.*, 1991). Reproductive decisions of this kind are complex, with social as well as individual implications. However, this is too often taken as a licence to remove a woman's freedom of choice on the grounds of presumed benefit to either herself, her unborn child or the wider society (Kass, 1991).

We have seen that women are increasingly vulnerable to contracting the HIV virus and often succumb to it more rapidly than their male counterparts. Evidence from around the world indicates that women have frequently been the focus of attention as potential transmitters of the disease, or as the moral guardians of their male partners. Yet many are denied access to appropriate preventive and curative services, especially in those parts of the world where their need is greatest. As the epidemic has progressed, women have taken increasing responsibility for those who are made sick or orphaned by AIDS. However, they have been allowed little influence over the relevant policy and planning decisions and have rarely had their own needs as people affected by HIV and AIDS taken seriously.

The Way Forward?

This global overview of the current situation of women in the AIDS pandemic offers a number of important lessons. While indicating the biological vulnerability shared by all women it also illustrates the specificity of the epidemics among women in different social contexts. While underlining the deep-seated male domination of heterosexuality it also identifies the variability of women's responses as they strive to meet their own needs and those of their families. But above all it demonstrates that in the absence of a vaccine, HIV and AIDS are not amenable to a simple technological 'fix'. No attempt to halt the heterosexual spread of AIDS will be successful unless it encompasses changes in the relations between the sexes on a scale as yet unprecedented. Indeed the pandemic itself offers women a unique opportunity to fight inequality and discrimination under the umbrella of better health for all.

If we are to seize this opportunity, women will need to be involved in all aspects of the development and implementation of strategies for both prevention and care. A number of international initiatives have now placed the needs of women firmly on the global agenda. In 1990, World AIDS Day focused on women and children, and a series of WHO conferences have suggested the broad outlines of a gendered strategy for HIV and AIDS (WHO, 1989a, 1989b). New initiatives are beginning to appear but much more work is needed at both national and local levels.

First, women must achieve greater control over their own sexuality. Health education can make a major contribution to this process if it is offered in accessible and culturally specific ways that are relevant to women's lives. Community-based projects often achieve the best results, enabling women to share their experiences and build up support networks in positive and unthreatening ways (Ulin, 1992). All over Africa, women are now working together on AIDS prevention work in projects of this kind (Berer with Ray, chapter 13).

Some of the most innovative schemes have been carried out among commercial sex workers. In Nairobi, for instance, members of a group who met together in highly interactive community meetings were twice as likely as those who did not attend to insist on condom use by their clients. Similarly positive results have been reported from groups of prostitute women in India, Thailand, Nigeria, Mexico and the Dominican Republic (de Bruyn, 1992; Berer with Ray, chapter 13).

In New York, the Brooklyn AIDS Task Force (BATF) helps Haitian women to develop prevention strategies through dealing with the problems they encounter in their everyday lives (Durand, 1990). Also in the United States, a number of inmates in Bedford Hills Correctional Facility came together to create AIDS Counselling and Education (ACE). At first they encountered considerable fear and hostility but their educational programme has made an impact on many women facing extremely difficult challenges (Women of ACE, Bedford Hills Correctional Facility). These small-scale experiments offer valuable examples of what can be achieved, and they need to be expanded to cover more groups of women. Even more importantly, similar techniques need to be used to persuade men too of the importance of changing to safer sex.

As well as education and community support, alternatives to the condom are urgently needed if women are to have the means to protect themselves. Safe and effective virucides could provide part of the answer, while the new female condom can potentially offer protection against both infection and pregnancy. Current trials of its effectiveness and acceptability show mixed results, and at present the cost is high but the device clearly has potential which needs further development (Liskin and Sakondhavat, 1992, p. 704).

In theory the female condom offers women their own barrier method that is at least as safe and effective as the male condom, yet preliminary studies show that in practice men can still have a major say in whether or not women protect themselves. In Kenya, men's objections were the main factor cited by the 40 per cent of commercial sex workers who abandoned the female condom after three weeks. Similarly, in a study in Cameroon more than 75 per cent of commercial sex workers had customers who refused to have intercourse if they used the female condom (Liskin and Sakondhavat, 1992). Thus technology alone will not solve the problem.

Attempts to enhance female sexual self-determination will need to give women greater control over all aspects of their lives, and better education and employment opportunities are central to this process.

25

Specific programmes to promote women's training have been developed among commercial sex workers in an attempt to offer them alternative ways of making a living. In Thailand, for example, the Empower Project offers bar hostesses health education programmes, a helpline, counselling and legal advice as well as teaching them marketable skills such as sewing and typing. Programmes of this kind are important for all those whose economic dependence makes them vulnerable to sexual and social pressures. Hence the active involvement of women in wider development strategies is an essential element in any effective HIV and AIDS prevention programme.

Alongside the empowerment gained through education and training, women also need equal access to comprehensive health services. This will contribute to their overall wellbeing as well as facilitating the identification and treatment of sexually transmitted diseases. For those women already affected by HIV and AIDS, health services need to be non-stigmatizing, with workers who respect their basic rights. An awareness of gender issues in both clinical and social research will be needed if more effective care is to be developed, while a greater awareness of women's psychosocial needs can ease their distress and optimize their quality of life.

2 Conclusion

The future pattern of HIV and AIDS in the UK remains uncertain, but there is already an epidemic among women in the third world. The flow of aid from the rich countries is already beginning to slow down and it is clear that many of the world's poorest women will be among the least visible and most numerous of those affected. This poses a major challenge for feminists of all nationalities. There is much we can learn about our own situation from those women already experiencing the effects of the epidemic. At the same time, we have a clear duty to support their efforts to limit the spread of HIV infection, not just in Britain but all over the world.

2 References

ALLEN, S., LINDAN, C., SERUFILIRA, A., VAN DE PERRE, P., CHEN RUNDLE, A., NSENGUMUREMYI, F., CARAEL, M., SCHWALBE, J. and HULLEY, S. (1993) 'HIV Infection in Childbearing Women in Kigali, Rwanda', In: BERER, M. with RAY, S.

(Eds) *Women and HIV/AIDS: An International Resource Book*, London, Pandora Press.

ANASTOS, K. and MARTE, C. (1991) 'Women — The Missing Persons in the AIDS Epidemic', In MCKENZIE, N. (Ed.) *The AIDS Reader: Social, Political and Ethical Issues*, Meridian.

ARAL, S. and HOLMES, K. (1991) 'Sexually Transmitted Diseases in the AIDS Era', *Scientific American*, 264:2, pp. 18–25.

BANG, R., BANG, A., BAITULE, M., CHOUDHARY, Y., SARMUKALAAM, S., and TALE, O. (1989) 'High Prevalence of Gynaecological Diseases in Rural Indian Women', *Lancet*, 19 Jan, pp. 85–8.

BANZHAF, M. (1990) 'Race, Women and AIDS: Introduction' In The ACT UP/New York Women and AIDS Book Group, *Women, AIDS and Activism*, Boston, South End Press.

BASSETT, M. and MHLOYI, M. (1991) 'Women and AIDS in Zimbabwe: The Making of an Epidemic', *International Journal of Health Services*, vol. 21, no. 1, pp. 143–56.

BERER, M. with RAY, S. (1993) *Women and HIV/AIDS: An International Resource Book*, London, Pandora Press.

BRETTLE, R. and LEEN, C. (1991) 'The Natural History of HIV and AIDS in Women', *AIDS*, vol. 5, pp. 1283–92.

CAROVANO, K. (1991) 'More than Mothers and Whores: Redefining the AIDS Prevention Needs of Women', *International Journal of Health Services*, vol. 21, no. 1, pp. 131–42.

COMMUNICABLE DISEASE REPORT (1993) vol. 3, no. 4. *AIDS and HIV in the United Kingdom: Monthly Report*, pp. 17–20.

DAVIS K. and ROWLAND, D. (1991) 'Uninsured and Undeserved: Inequities in Health Care in the United States', In MCKENZIE, N. (Ed.) *The AIDS Reader: Social, Political and Ethical Issues*, Meridian.

DE BRUYN, M. (1992) 'Women and AIDS in Developing Countries', *Social Science and Medicine*, vol. 34, no. 3, pp. 249–62.

DENENBERG, R. (1990a) 'Treatment and Trials', In The ACT UP/NEW YORK Women and AIDS Book Group *Women, AIDS and Activism*, Boston, South End Press.

DENENBERG, R. (1990b) 'Unique Aspects of HIV Infection in Women', In THE ACT UP/ NEW YORK WOMEN AND AIDS BOOK GROUP *Women, AIDS and Activism*, Boston, South End Press.

DURAND, Y. (1990) 'Cultural Sensitivity in Practice' In THE ACT UP/NEW YORK WOMEN AND AIDS BOOK GROUP *Women, AIDS and Activism*, Boston, South End Press.

FADEN, R., GELLER, G. and POWERS, M. (Eds) (1991) *AIDS, Women and the Next Generation: Towards a Morally Acceptable Public Policy for HIV Testing of Pregnant Women and Newborns*, Oxford, Oxford University Press.

FORD, N. and KOETSAWANG, S. (1991) 'The Sociocultural Context of the Transmission of HIV in Thailand', *Social Science and Medicine*, vol. 33, no. 4, pp. 405–14.

FOUCAULT, M. (1978) *The History of Sexuality*, Harmondsworth, Penguin.

GRUNDFEST SCHOEPF, B., ENGUNDU, W., WA NKERA, R., NTSOMO, P. and SCHOEPF, C. (1991) 'Gender, Power and Risk of AIDS in Zaire' In TURSHEN, M. (Ed.) *Women and Health in Africa*, Trenton, NJ, Africa World Press.

HATCHER, R., KOWAL, D., GUEST, F., TUNSSELL, J., STEWART, F., STEWART, G., BOWN, S. and CATES, W. (1989) *Contraceptive Technology: International Edition*, Atlanta Georgia, Printed Matter.

HOLLAND, J., RAMAZANOGLU, C., SCOTT, S., SHARPE, S. and THOMSON, R. (1990) 'Sex, Gender and Power: Young Women's Sexuality in the Shadow of AIDS', *Sociology of Health and Illness*, vol. 12, no. 3, pp. 336–50.

JACOBSON, J. (1992) 'Women's Health: The Price of Poverty', In KOBLINKSY, M., TIMYAN, J. and GAY, J. (Eds) (1992) *The Health of Women: A Global Perspective*, Boulder, Colorado, Westview Press.

JOCHELSON, K., MOTHIBELI, M. and LEGER, J-P. (1991) 'Human Immunodeficiency Virus and Migrant Labour in South Africa', *International Journal of Health Services*, vol. 21, no. 1, pp. 157–73.

KASS, N. (1991) 'Reproductive Decision Making in the Context of HIV: The Case for Nondirective Counselling', In FADEN, R., GELLER, G. and POWERS, M. (Eds) *AIDS, Women and the Next Generation: Towards a Morally Acceptable Public Policy for HIV Testing of Pregnant Women and Newborns*, Oxford, Oxford University Press.

KISEKKA, M.N. (1990) 'AIDS in Uganda as a Gender Issue', In ROTHBLUM, E. and COLE, E. (Eds) *Women's Mental Health in Africa*, New York, Harrington Park Press.

KLINE, A., KLINE, E. and OKEN, E. (1992) 'Minority Women and Sexual Choice in the Age of AIDS', *Social Science and Medicine*, vol. 34, no. 4, pp. 447–57.

KYNCH, T. and SEN, A. (1983) 'Indian Women: Wellbeing and Survival', *Cambridge Journal of Economics*, vol. 7, pp. 363–80.

LAGA, M. (1992) 'Human Immunodeficiency Virus Infection Prevention: The Need for Complementary STD Control', In GERMAIN, A., HOLMES, K. PIOT, P. and WASSERHEIT, J. (Eds) *Reproductive Tract Infections: Global Impact and Priorities for Women's Reproductive Health*, New York, Plenum Press.

LISKIN, L., and SAKONDHAVAT, C. (1992) 'The Female Condom: A New Option for Women', In MANN, J., TARANTOLA, D. and NETTER, T. (Eds) *AIDS in the World: A Global Report*, Harvard University Press, pp. 700–7.

MANN, J., TARANTOLA, D. and NETTER, T. (1992) *AIDS in the World: A Global Report*, Harvard University Press.

MARTE, C. (1992) 'Cervical Cancer', In MANN, J., TARANTOLA, D., and NETTER, T. (1992) *AIDS in the World: A Global Report*, Harvard University Press.

OFFICE OF RESEARCH ON WOMEN'S HEALTH (1992) *Report of the National Institutes of Health: Opportunities for Research on Women's Health, September 1991, Hunt Valley, Md*, US National Institutes of Health, Washington DC.

O'SULLIVAN, S. and THOMSON, K. (1992) *Positively Women: Living with AIDS*, London, Sheba Feminist Press.

PANOS INSTITUTE (1990) *Triple Jeopardy: Women and AIDS*, London, Panos Publications.

PANOS INSTITUTE (1992) *The Hidden Cost of AIDS: The Challenge of HIV to Development*, London, Panos Publications.

RAVINDRAN, S. (1986) *Health Implications of Sex Discrimination in Childhood: A Review Paper and Annotated Bibliography*, Geneva, WHO/UNICEF, 86.2

REID, E. (1992) 'Gender, Knowledge and Responsibility', In MANN, J., TARANTOLA, D. and NETTER, T. (1992) *AIDS in the World: A Global Report*, Harvard University Press.

RICHARDSON, D. (1987) *Women and the AIDS Crisis*, London, Pandora Press.

ROSSER, S. (1992) 'Revisioning Clinical Research: Gender and the Ethics of Experimental Design', In BEQUAERT HOLMES, H. and PURDY, L. (Eds) *Feminist Perspectives in Medical Ethics*, Indiana University Press.

ROTHENBERG, R., WOELFEL, M., STONEBURNER, R., MILBERG, T., PARKER, R. and TRUMAN, B. (1987) 'Survival with the Acquired Immune Deficiency Syndrome', *New England Journal of Medicine*, vol. 317, no. 21, pp. 1297–1302.

SEIDEL, G. (1993) 'The Competing Discourses of HIV/AIDS in Sub-Saharan Africa: Discourses of Rights and Empowerment vs Discourses of Control and Exclusion', *Social Science and Medicine*, vol. 36, no. 3, pp. 175–94.

ULIN, P. (1992) 'African Women and AIDS: Negotiating Behavioural Change', *Social Science and Medicine*, vol. 34, no. 1, pp. 63–73.

WALKER, J. (1990) 'Women and Children', In THE ACT UP/NEW YORK WOMEN AND AIDS BOOK GROUP, *Women, AIDS and Activism*, Boston, South End Press.

WASSERHEIT, T. and HOLMES, K. (1992) 'Reproductive Tract Infections: Challenges for International Health Policy, Programs and Research, In GERMAIN, A., HOLMES, K., PIOT, P. and WASSERHEIT, J. (Eds) *Reproductive Tract Infections: Global Impact and Priorities for Women's Reproductive Health,* New York, Plenum Press.

WEEKS, J. (1986) *Sexuality,* London, Tavistock/Chichester, Ellis Horwood.

WILKINSON, S. and KITZINGER, C. (1993) *Heterosexuality: A Feminism and Psychology Reader,* London, Sage Publications.

WORLD HEALTH ORGANIZATION (1989a) *Report of the Consultation with International Women's NGOs on AIDS Prevention and Care,* Geneva, WHO Global Programme on AIDS.

WORLD HEALTH ORGANIZATION (1989b) *Report of the Meeting on Research Priorities Relating to Women and HIV/AIDS,* Geneva, WHO Global Programme on AIDS.

WORLD HEALTH ORGANIZATION (1992) *Women's Health: Across Age and Frontier,* Geneva, WHO.

WORTH, D. (1989) 'Sexual Decision Making and AIDS: Why Condom Promotion among Vulnerable Women Is Likely to Fail' *Studies in Family Planning,* vol. 20, no. 6, pp. 297-367.

ZWI, A. and CABRAL, A. (1991) 'Identifying High Risk Situations for Preventing AIDS', *British Medical Journal,* 303, pp. 1527-9.

Chapter 2

Women and HIV/AIDS: Medical Issues

Judy Bury

For the first few years of the AIDS epidemic, AIDS was seen as a disease affecting only gay men. By 1985, however, it was clear that, even in the developed countries, people other than gay men were developing AIDS — people who had become infected through blood transfusions, through sharing needles or through heterosexual intercourse. AIDS was also seen in babies born to women who had been infected heterosexually or through needle sharing. Not only men but also women and children were developing AIDS and the fact that women were at risk could no longer be ignored. But as women became infected and began to look for information and support, they found that the information available often did not apply to women, that most services had been established by men for men, and that doctors and other professionals were often unprepared for the particular issues that women would raise.

Once it became clear that women were at risk from AIDS, one of the first questions asked was about the implications of AIDS for childbearing. This is an important question and one where the information given to women has often been misleading or worse. But the ability to bear children is not the only factor that distinguishes women from men and, as the epidemic has progressed, it has become clear that there are many other medical questions to which women need answers: are women more likely to be infected heterosexually than men, and if so, why? can HIV infection be transmitted during lesbian sex? do HIV disease and AIDS take a different form in women compared with men? This chapter attempts to answer some of these questions.

Women and Heterosexual Transmission

The risk of HIV infection being transmitted heterosexually has been one of many issues around HIV and AIDS that is associated with confusion

30

and prejudice. It has been obvious at least since the mid 1980s that HIV infection can be transmitted through heterosexual sex, yet there are those who continue to talk about the myth of heterosexual transmission. And some of the same people who claim that the risk of heterosexual transmission is exaggerated, talk about the danger of prostitutes infecting their clients or make much of the fact that many of those who have become infected heterosexually have been infected abroad. These statements all serve to fuel the idea that HIV infection only infects 'other' people — that is, people other than white, heterosexual, non-drug-users. But these beliefs are also related to an attempt to blame 'other' people for the spread of HIV infection. Thus, gay men, Africans, drug users and prostitutes have all been blamed, while they are often contrasted with 'innocent' victims of the epidemic such as recipients of infected blood or blood products, and HIV-infected babies. Such confusion and prejudice have often made it difficult for women (and men) to find out the facts about heterosexual transmission.

In fact, there is no doubt at all that HIV infection can be transmitted heterosexually. In order for sexual transmission to occur, infected blood, semen or vaginal fluid has to find its way in the bloodstream. Although HIV has been isolated from other fluids such as saliva, urine and faeces, the virus is not present in sufficient amounts in these fluids to cause infection, even if these fluids get into the bloodstream of an uninfected person.

Although HIV is poorly transmitted during sexual intercourse compared with other sexually transmitted diseases such as gonorrhoea (Alexander, 1990) some people have become infected after a single act of sexual intercourse (see e.g. Johnson, 1988). It seems that some people are more infectious than others and that some people are more susceptible to infection than others (Bury, 1989) which makes it impossible to give a figure for the risk of contracting HIV infection from one sexual exposure.

There is some evidence that men with HIV infection are approximately twice as likely to infect their female sexual partners as women with HIV infection are to infect their male partners, but there is no doubt that both can happen (Alexander, 1990; Johnson, 1990).

A person with HIV infection may infect his or her sexual partner during vaginal or anal intercourse at any time, although they are more likely to do so at the time of seroconversion and later on in the disease as they become ill. People with HIV infection are also more likely to infect their partner if either has genital ulceration or genital warts (Alexander, 1990).

The risk of transmitting HIV infection during kissing or oral sex is very small — there have been only a handful of cases reported worldwide and in all instances it seems that the virus entered the bloodstream of the uninfected partner through sores or ulcers in the mouth.

The fact that women are more at risk from heterosexual transmission than men has not prevented women from being held responsible or even blamed for heterosexual transmission. Prostitutes are blamed even when their clients pay extra for unprotected sex; in many of the prevention campaigns, the emphasis has been on persuading women that it is their responsibility to ensure that men use condoms; and in one of the early British campaigns, women were represented as beautiful temptresses who might be HIV 'carriers'.

The Risks of Lesbian Sex

The risk of HIV transmission through most lesbian sexual activities is very small (Chu, *et al.*, 1990a). There have been only a few cases reported worldwide and they were all cases in which there had been sexual activity involving blood. Undoubtedly there is underreporting of lesbian sexual transmission as many lesbian women may be reluctant to acknowledge their sexual orientation to their doctor. In order for infection to occur, infected vaginal fluid or blood (including menstrual blood) would have to get into the bloodstream through cuts or sores in the vulva, vagina, mouth or skin. Thus, although HIV transmission through lesbian sex seems to be uncommon, lesbian sex is not without risk as was thought at first and there have been significant moves in the lesbian community to emphasize that 'low risk isn't no risk'.

Apart from the few lesbians who have become infected through lesbian sex, there are many others who have become infected through intercourse with a man, through sharing needles or as a result of artificial insemination. In other words, we are put at risk by what we do, not by how we define ourselves or who we are.

The Risks of Pregnancy and Childbearing

The risks of pregnancy and childbearing for women with HIV infection is another area where confusion has resulted from prejudice but, in this case, also from wrong information. Early uncontrolled studies suggested that pregnancy was dangerous for women with AIDS and also suggested that the risk of the baby being infected was high (50 to 60 per cent) (Bury, 1992). Although these studies have now been superseded, their impact remains. There continue to be reports of women being advised not to become pregnant or to have their pregnancy terminated because of the risk to their health. Women are also given misleading information about the possibility that their baby will be infected.

Women with HIV infection contemplating pregnancy need information about four main issues: the effect of pregnancy on the progression of HIV disease; the effect of HIV infection on the outcome of pregnancy; the risk of materno-foetal transmission of HIV infection; and the risk of breast-feeding.

Pregnancy and the Progression of HIV Disease

Over the last five years evidence has accumulated to suggest that pregnancy does not affect the progression of HIV disease for women who are still asymptomatic and whose immune system is still intact (MacCallum *et al.*, 1988; Schoenbaum *et al.*, 1988). However, once the disease has progressed to the stage where the woman's immune system has been compromised and especially if she already has HIV-related symptoms, pregnancy may cause more rapid progression of the disease. Although recent studies have been reassuring about the risks of pregnancy, it has been pointed out (Minkoff, 1987) that pregnancy may still involve some dangers for a woman with HIV infection as pregnancy may mask the early symptoms of HIV disease such as tiredness and breathlessness. In addition, if a woman develops AIDS during pregnancy, treatment may be more difficult as some of the useful drugs might harm the foetus.

HIV Infection and the Outcome of Pregnancy

A number of studies have found that women with HIV infection who remain well fare no worse during their pregnancies than women in similar circumstances who were not HIV infected (Johnstone *et al.*, 1988; Selwyn *et al.*, 1989). European studies suggest that asymptomatic HIV infection does not seem to increase the risk of having a miscarriage, a stillbirth, a premature baby or a baby of low birthweight. However, some African studies suggest that symptomatic HIV disease may be associated with an increased risk of miscarriage, prematurity, or low birthrate (Johnstone, 1993).

The Risk of Materno-Foetal Transmission

HIV infection can pass from a mother to her baby during pregnancy or at the time of delivery. Although vaginal delivery may increase the risk of transmission (Chiodo *et al.*, 1986), it is still not clear whether Caesarian section would protect the foetus from infection (Mok, 1993).

At present it is not possible to test reliably for the virus itself, so the diagnosis of HIV infection depends on the presence of HIV antibodies. All infants born to HIV-positive mothers will have HIV antibodies (maternal antibodies) at birth. These antibodies clear by 18 months so that if a baby is not infected, it will be HIV negative by 18 months. If the baby is infected, it will make its own antibodies to HIV, thus remaining HIV-positive beyond 18 months. Thus it is not possible to know whether or not a baby is infected until it is 18 months of age. Other tests that may allow earlier diagnosis are being evaluated but are not yet available (Peckham and Newell, 1990). In a recent study of 600 babies born to HIV-infected mothers in ten European Centres, only 13 per cent had persistent HIV antibodies after 18 months, suggesting a transmission rate of approximately one in eight, much lower than previously thought (European Collaborative Study, 1991).

One important factor that seems to affect the risk of materno-foetal transmission is the health of the mother during pregnancy. In one study, infants born to mothers who had symptoms of HIV infection during pregnancy were nine times more likely to develop AIDS or AIDS-related complex than infants of mothers who were clinically well during pregnancy (Mok *et al.*, 1987). It has been suggested that there may also be a greater risk of transmission at the time that a woman becomes HIV-antibody-positive (seroconversion) — a time when there are large numbers of the HIV in the bloodstream. Although this is still uncertain, this possibility has implications for those advising women without HIV infection but who have an HIV-positive partner and who risk becoming infected at the time of conception or during the pregnancy.

Breast-Feeding

There have been a few reported cases of postnatal transmission of HIV infection from an infected mother to her baby via breast milk, usually in cases where the mother acquired the infection from a blood transfusion given postnatally. One study (Ziegler *et al.*, 1988) suggests that the risk is greatest if the mother seroconverts while she is breast-feeding, perhaps due to the presence of large numbers of the HIV in the blood at that time.

As already discussed, it is not possible to be certain whether a baby is infected until some months after birth. A recent study suggests that breast feeding may increase the risk of HIV transmission to the baby (European Collaborative Study, 1992), so HIV-infected mothers need to be informed about the possible risk. In countries such as Britain and the US where safe alternatives to breast-feeding are available, they may choose not to breast-feed. In countries where safe alternatives to breast-feeding may not be available, the additional risk of infection from breast-feeding may be less than the dangers to the baby's health of not breast-feeding. Women at high risk of infection (those still injecting drugs or partners of men with HIV infection) should also be informed of the potential risks of breast-feeding.

Counselling HIV-Positive Women about Pregnancy

It is now possible for a woman to be given more individual advice about the risk of pregnancy for her and her baby. If a woman has symptoms of HIV infection or has AIDS there is a substantial risk that the baby will be infected and that pregnancy will cause a more rapid progression of her illness. If she is asymptomatic, immunological and virological blood tests might give some clues about disease progression and the likelihood of imminent clinical deterioration (Anonymous, 1988). If there is no evidence of severe damage to the immune system and clinical deterioration does not seem imminent, and if she is keen to have a baby, even knowing that the baby might be infected, it is probably better for her to have a baby sooner rather than later, as her health is less likely to be affected, the baby is less likely to be infected, and she is likely to have more years to spend with the baby before becoming ill herself.

In summary, pregnancy does not seem to be dangerous for women with HIV infection as long as they remain well and the risk of the baby being infected may be less than was thought. On the basis of immunological and virological tests, women may be offered individual advice about the risk of pregnancy to them and to their baby. Women with HIV infection or at high risk of infection need information about the potential risks of breast-feeding.

The Physical Effects of HIV Disease on Women

HIV infection mostly follows the same pattern in men and women. Between a few days and a few months after infection, around the time that the HIV antibody test becomes positive, there may be a short illness like flu or glandular fever (Leen and Brettle, 1991). This 'seroconversion illness' is only experienced by a minority of those who become infected.

People with HIV infection then remain well for some years before developing symptoms of HIV disease. Early symptoms include enlarged lymph nodes, weight loss, fevers, sweats and diarrhoea. This combination of symptoms is sometimes known as AIDS-related complex (ARC) although this term is being used less and less. As HIV infection continues to damage the immune system, the body is less able to defend itself against infections (known as opportunistic infections) and cancer. AIDS (acquired immune deficiency syndrome) is diagnosed once one of a number of conditions has developed, such as *Pneumocystis carinii* pneumonia (PCP) or Kaposi's sarcoma (KS), that indicate severe immune damage. These conditions are defined by the Centers for Disease Control in Atlanta, Georgia in the US. Studies on gay men suggest that on average it takes ten years for someone with HIV infection to develop AIDS (e.g. Moss and Bacchetti, 1989; Rutherford *et al.*, 1990); that is, 50 per cent of men will develop AIDS within ten years of infection with HIV while 50 per cent of men with HIV infection will take longer than ten years to develop AIDS. Similar research has not been done on drug users or on women with HIV infection so at the present time it is not possible to say how long it takes for a woman with HIV infection to develop AIDS. This in part depends on whether women develop the same 'AIDS-defining illnesses' that are found in men.

Women experience the same spectrum of illnesses associated with AIDS apart from Kaposi's sarcoma (KS). This slowly progressing skin cancer, which is a common manifestation of AIDS in men, seems to be a sexually transmitted condition (Beral *et al.*, 1990) which is only rarely seen in those who have acquired HIV infection through needle sharing (Leen and Brettle, 1991). Women who have acquired HIV infection heterosexually are more likely to have KS if their partners are bisexual men than if they are injecting drug users (Beral *et al.*, 1990) and women may also develop KS if they have become infected by a blood transfusion (Lassoued *et al.*, 1991). Although uncommon in women, when it does develop it may spread more rapidly than in men and can be fatal (*ibid.*). In men with HIV infection, KS is often the first condition to occur that indicates that the man has AIDS and it may occur a long time before other AIDS-defining conditions. As women rarely develop KS, their diagnosis of AIDS almost always depends on the appearance of other conditions such as pneumocystis pneumonia which usually appear later in the disease.

People with HIV disease are particularly prone to infections with candida (thrush). In men or women this can affect the mouth or oesophagus (gullet) and in women it can also affect the vagina. Vaginal thrush (candidiasis) is very common in women with HIV infection

(Rhoads *et al.*, 1987). It often recurs after treatment and may become severe and unresponsive to treatment as HIV disease progresses (Brettle and Leen, 1991).

Women with HIV infection are also more likely to develop other gynaecological infections. Genital warts, genital herpes and pelvic inflammatory disease are all common in women with HIV infection and, like thrush, they may be recurrent and severe (Brettle and Leen, 1991). Once the immune system has been severely damaged, a woman's body may not be able to respond to an infection with pain and inflammation so that the diagnosis may be missed. Continuing untreated infection may then cause further damage to the immune system.

Women with HIV infection have been found to be more likely to develop abnormal cervical smears (cervical dysplasia) and possibly cervical cancer, apparently related to the increased incidence of genital herpes infection (Centers for Disease Control, 1990). Continuing immune damage is associated with increasing abnormalities of cervical cells (Brettle and Leen, 1991). It is interesting to note that there has been no increase in the incidence of cervical cancer in New York, and cervical cancer is rarely listed as a cause of HIV-related death. Nevertheless, it is advisable for women with HIV infection to be offered regular and frequent (at least annual) cervical smears.

As discussed previously, the diagnosis of AIDS depends on the appearance of one of a number of conditions that are defined by the Centers for Disease Control (CDC). Although this list of conditions was broadened in 1987, until 1993 it did not include any of the gynaecological conditions that are associated with HIV infection in women. Thus many women died from HIV-associated conditions without a diagnosis of AIDS. In a study of deaths of women with HIV/AIDS in the US it was found that 48 per cent died of conditions not listed in the CDC definition for AIDS (Chu *et al.*, 1990b). A great deal of pressure was put on the CDC to include gynaecological conditions in the list of AIDS-defining diagnoses (ACT UP, 1991) but they resisted for some time, giving as their main reason that none of these conditions are specific to women with HIV infection.

The exclusion of gynaecological conditions from the current definition of AIDS has a number of results. Firstly, women are underrepresented in AIDS statistics. Secondly, in countries such as the US where certain benefits are only available once someone has an AIDS diagnosis, many women with severe HIV disease will not be eligible for benefits. Thirdly, many women with severe HIV disease are excluded from trials of new drugs, as some of these are only given to those with an AIDS diagnosis. In 1993, the CDC partially relented, adding three more conditions, including cervical dysplasia, to the list of AIDS-defining conditions.

Survival of Women with AIDS

A number of studies of survival of people with AIDS have found that women survive a significantly shorter time after a diagnosis of AIDS than men (e.g. Rothenberg *et al.*, 1987) and black women drug users survive the shortest time of all (*ibid.*). Over the last few years men and women have been living longer after a diagnosis of AIDS but in studies in the UK and the US women still survive for a shorter time than men (Lemp *et al.*, 1990; Willocks *et al.*, 1991).

Shorter survival in women could be due to a number of factors. AIDS sometimes takes a much slower course in men who present with Kaposi's Sarcoma which is a rare presentation in women (see above). Women tend to come forward later in the disease than men, particularly in the US where they have poorer access to health care due to poverty (Springer, 1992). Poor minority women in particular are unlikely to be receiving ongoing preventive medical care and may be reluctant to seek help when they are ill. Women may also be slow to come forward because they consider their own health needs after the needs of their family. Doctors may contribute to the poor survival of women as they are sometimes slow to recognize symptoms of AIDS when they present in women and may give them inappropriate treatment (Springer, 1992). In addition, women are less likely to be offered new drug treatments (see below). Another possible explanation for shorter survival could be biological differences between men and women in disease progression (ACT UP, 1991).

A recent study in Edinburgh controlled for a number of these factors by comparing the progression of HIV infection in male and female drug users of similar background where all had been receiving good medical care. Even here male drug users were found to survive significantly longer after a diagnosis of AIDS than female drug users (Willocks *et al.*, 1991). The authors commented that many of the women are principal carers for children 'and thus may receive less prophylactic and pre-AIDS care' (*ibid.*).

There is clearly a need for more research into HIV disease in women. A new study being carried out in the UK is designed to look at the natural history of HIV infection and AIDS in women. Early drafts of the research protocol included questions about sociodemographic factors which would have allowed an assessment of the extent to which these might contribute to different survival patterns in women compared to men but most of these questions have been omitted from the final protocol, apparently due to lack of funding.

Women, Drug Trials and Research

There are very few drugs that have been approved for the treatment of HIV disease and AIDS. Many new drugs are under trial and for some people with HIV disease, the only access to drug treatment may be to take part in the trial of a new drug. Yet, much research on new drugs for HIV disease is limited to men. Even women with an AIDS diagnosis are often excluded from drug trials for fear that they may become pregnant during the treatment and that the drug might damage the foetus. They are only included in trials of some drugs if they are using 'adequate birth control' which sometimes requires sterilization (ACT UP, 1991).

Some drug trials do include women but the trial design rarely includes questions about the effect of the drug on menstruation, or on the progression of gynaecological conditions such as vaginal thrush, pelvic infection or cervical cancer (ACT UP, 1991). Some women have noticed that drugs used for the treatment of AIDS such as AZT (Zidovudine) and ddI can cause painful, heavy and prolonged periods but these effects have not been studied (ACT UP, 1991).

HIV/AIDS is still a relatively new disease and a great deal of research has been and is being conducted in order to understand more about the various manifestations of HIV infection and AIDS. Women are clearly underrepresented in this research (ACT UP, 1991) and although some researchers (e.g. Brettle and Leen, 1991) recognize that there is a lack of knowledge about the course of HIV infection and AIDS in women, women are still being excluded from much of the relevant research (ACT UP, 1991). As women are increasingly affected by HIV and AIDS, this becomes increasingly inexcusable.

References

ACT UP (1991) *Treatment and Research Agenda for Women with HIV Infection*, US, AIDS Coalition to Unleash Power.
ALEXANDER, N.J. (1990) 'Sexual Transmission of Human Immunodeficiency Virus: Virus Entry into the Male and Female Genital Tract', *Fertility and Sterility*, vol. 54, no. 1, pp. 1-18.

ANONYMOUS (1988) 'HIV Infection: Obstetric and Perinatal Issues', *Lancet,* vol. 1, 9 April, pp. 806-7.

BERAL, V., PETERMAN, T.A., BERKELMAN, R.L. and JAFFE, H.W. (1990) 'Kaposi's sarcoma among Persons with AIDS: A Sexually Transmitted Infection?' *Lancet,* vol. 335, 20 Jan, pp. 123-8.

BRETTLE, R.P. and LEEN, C.L.S. (1991) 'The Natural History of HIV and AIDS in Women', *AIDS,* 5, pp. 1283-92.

BURY, J. (1989) 'Counselling Women with HIV Infection about Pregnancy, Heterosexual Transmission and Contraception', *British Journal of Family Planning,* 14, pp. 116-22.

BURY, J. (1992) 'Pregnancy, Heterosexual Transmission and Contraception', In BURY, J., MORRISON, V. and MCLACHLAN, S. (Eds) *Working with Women and AIDS,* London, Routledge.

CENTERS FOR DISEASE CONTROL (1990) 'Risk for Cervical Disease in HIV-Infected Women — New York City', *Morbidity and Mortality Weekly Report,* 39 (47) pp. 846-9.

CHIODO, F., RICCHI, E., COSTIGLIOLA, P., MICHELACCI, L., BOVICELLI, L. and DALLACASA, P. (1986), 'Vertical Transmission of HTLV-III', *Lancet,* vol. 1, 29 March, p. 739.

CHU, S.Y., BUEHLER, J.W., FLEMING, P.L. and BERKELMAN, R.L. (1990a) 'Epidemiology of Reported Cases of AIDS in Lesbians, United States, 1980-89', *American Journal of Public Health,* 80, pp. 1380-1.

CHU, S.Y., BUEHLER, J.W. and BERKELMAN, R.L. (1990b) 'Impact of the Human Immunodeficiency Virus Epidemic on Mortality in Women of Reproductive Age, United States', *Journal of the American Medical Association,* 264 (2), pp. 225-9.

EUROPEAN COLLABORATIVE STUDY (1991) 'Children Born to Women with HIV-1 Infection: Natural History and Risk of Transmission', *Lancet,* 337, pp. 253-60.

EUROPEAN COLLABORATIVE STUDY (1992) 'Risk factors for mother-to-child transmission of HIV-1', *Lancet,* 339, pp. 1007-12.

JOHNSON, A.M. (1988) 'Heterosexual Transmission of Human Immunodeficiency Virus', *British Medical Journal,* vol. 296, 9 April, pp. 1017-20.

JOHNSON, A. (1990) 'The Epidemiology of HIV in the UK: Sexual Transmission', In HEALTH DEPARTMENTS AND HEALTH EDUCATION AUTHORITY, *HIV and AIDS: An Assessment of Current and Future Spread in the UK,* UK London, HMSO.

JOHNSTONE, F.D. (1993) 'Pregnancy in HIV-infected women'. In JOHNSTONE, M. and JOHNSTONE, F.D. (Eds), *HIV Infection in Women,* Edinburgh, Churchill Livingstone.

JOHNSTONE, F.D., MACCALLUM, L. BRETTLE, R., INGLIS, J.M. and PEUTHERER, J.F. (1988) 'Does Infection with HIV Affect the Outcome of Pregnancy?, *British Medical Journal,* Vol. 296, 13 February, p. 467.

LASSOUED, K., CLAUVEL, J-P., FEGUEUX, S., MATHERON, S., GORIN, I. and OKSENHENDLER, E. (1991) 'AIDS-Associated Kaposi's Sarcoma in Female Patients', *AIDS,* 5, pp. 877-80.

LEEN, C.L.S. and BRETTLE, R.P. (1991) 'Natural History of HIV Infection' In BIRD, G. (Ed.) *Immunology of HIV Infection,* London, Kluwer Press.

LEMP, G.F., PAYNE, S.F., NEAL, D. *et al.,* (1990) 'Survival Trends for Patients with AIDS', *Journal of the American Medical Association,* Vol. 263(3), pp. 402-6.

LIFSON, A.R. and ROGERS, M.R. (1986) 'Vertical Transmission of Human Immunodeficiency Virus', *Lancet,* vol. II, 9 August, p. 337.

MACCALLUM, L.R., FRANCE, A.J., JONES, M.E., STEEL, C.M., BURNS, S.M. and BRETTLE, R.P. (1988) 'The Effect of Pregnancy on the Progression of HIV Infection', paper presented at IVth International Conference on AIDS, Stockholm.

MINKOFF, H.L. (1987) 'Care of Pregnant Women Infected with Human Immunodeficiency Virus', *Journal of the American Medical Association*, vol. 258, pp. 2714–7.

MOK, J.Y.Q. (1993) 'Vertical transmission'. In JOHNSTONE, M. and JOHNSTONE, F.D. (Eds), *HIV Infection in Women*, Edinburgh, Churchill Livingstone.

MOK, J.Q., GIAQUINTO, C. DE ROSSI, A., GROSCH-WÖRNER, I., ADES, A.E. and PECKHAM, C.S. (1987) 'Infants Born to Mothers Seropositive for Human Immunodeficiency Virus', *Lancet*, vol. 1, 23 May, pp. 1164–7.

MOSS, A.R. and BACCHETTI, P. (1989) 'Natural History of HIV Infection', *AIDS*, 3, pp. 55–61.

PECKHAM, C.S. and NEWELL, M-L. (1990) 'HIV-1 Infection in Mothers and Babies', *AIDS Care*, vol. 2, no. 3, pp. 205–11.

RHOADS, J.L., WRIGHT, C., REDFIELD, R.R. *et al.* (1987) 'Chronic Vaginal Candidiasis in Women with Human Immunodeficiency Virus Infection', *Journal of the American Medical Association*, vol. 257, pp. 3105–7.

ROTHENBERG, R., WOELFEL, M., STONEBURNER, R. *et al.* (1987) 'Survival with the Acquired Immunodeficiency Syndrome', *New England Journal of Medicine*, 317, pp. 1297–302.

RUTHERFORD, G.W., LIFSON, A.R., HESSOL, N.A. *et. al.,* (1990) 'Course of HIV-1 Infection in a Cohort of Homosexual and Bisexual Men: An 11 Year Follow Up Study', *British Medical Journal*, vol. 301, 24 November, pp. 1183–8.

SCHOENBAUM, E.E., DAVENNY, K. and SELWYN, P.A. (1988) 'The Impact of Pregnancy on HIV-Related Disease', In HUDSON, C. and SHARP, F. (Eds) *AIDS and Obstetrics and Gynaecology*, London, Royal College of Obstetricians and Gynaecologists.

SELWYN, P.A., SCHOENBAUM, E.E., DAVENNY, K., ROBERTSON, V.J., FEINGOLD, A.R., SHULMAN, J.F., MAYERS, M.M., KLEIN, R.S., FRIEDLAND, G.H. and ROGERS, M.F. (1989) 'Prospective Study of Human Immunodeficiency Virus Infection and Pregnancy Outcome in Intravenous Drug Users', *Journal of the American Medical Association*, vol. 261, no. 9, pp. 1289–94.

SPRINGER, F. (1992) 'Some Reflections on Women with HIV/AIDS in New York City and the US', In BURY, J., MORRISON, V. and MCLACHLAN, S. (Eds), *Working with Women and AIDS*, London, Routledge.

WILLOCKS, L., COWAN, S.M., BRETTLE, R.P., MACCALLUM, L.R., MCHARDY, S. and RICHARDSON, A. (1991) 'Natural History of Early HIV Infection in Scottish Women', paper presented at VIIth International Conference on AIDS, Florence.

ZIEGLER, J.B., STEWART, G.J., PENNY, R., STUCKEY, M. and GOOD, S. (1988) 'Breast Feeding and Transmission of HIV from Mother to Infant', paper presented at IVth International Conference on AIDS, Stockholm.

Chapter 3

AIDS: Issues for Feminism in the UK

Diane Richardson

AIDS Is a Women's Issue

Although there is a vast literature on HIV/AIDS, relatively little has been written about how HIV/AIDS affects women. In part, this reflects the way AIDS was initially perceived in the West as a 'men's disease', so much so that until a few years ago a common response to attempts to discuss the topic of women and AIDS was 'Do women get AIDS?', the assumption being that women were at little or no risk. This assumption is contradicted by research findings and reported figures. In recent years it has become increasingly clear that women can both become infected with HIV and transmit the virus. In the UK, although the number of women who are HIV-positive is still low in global terms, the pattern of infection is of growing concern. Cases of AIDS among women have increased rapidly, by 51% in the two consecutive twelve-month periods, January 1992–December 1993 (from 142 to 215); 19% of all those reported to be HIV positive in that period are women (Communicable Disease Surveillance Centre figures to the end of December 1993).

Much of the published work on women and AIDS, especially medical and scientific publications, has concentrated on women as carers of people with AIDS or as possible transmittors of the HIV virus, with the focus largely on prostitutes and pregnant women. The underlying concern would seem to be how to protect the health of men and children, rather than addressing women's health needs. Of the limited amount of work which does address the issues HIV/AIDS raises for women, some concentrates primarily on providing practical information about HIV/AIDS and advice on prevention, with different authors favouring different risk-reduction strategies. (Contrast, for example, the somewhat moralistic advice offered by Helen Kaplan (1987) with the approach taken by Cindy Patton and Janis Kelly (1987).) Other contributions to work on women and AIDS have attempted to discuss not only the range of HIV/AIDS issues affecting women specifically, but also to acknowledge the wider social context of AIDS prevention, diagnosis and treatment (e.g. Richardson, 1987; Panos Institute, 1990; Patton, 1993). There have, in addition, been a number of books published consisting largely of personal accounts by women living with HIV or AIDS and/or who are involved in AIDS work (e.g. Rieder and Ruppelt, 1989; O'Sullivan and Thomson, 1992; Rudd and Taylor, 1992).

The year 1987 was an important one in terms of public recognition of AIDS as a women's health issue. Prior to then, there had been very little written about women and AIDS. However, 1987 saw the publication of a number of books: for example, in the United States, Chris Norwood's *Advice for Life: A Woman's Guide to AIDS Risks and Prevention,* Helen Singer Kaplan's (awful) *The Real Truth About Women and AIDS: How to Eliminate the Risks Without Giving Up Love and Sex,* and Cindy Patton and Janis Kelly's *Making It: A Women's Guide to Sex in the Age of AIDS.* In Britain my own book *Women and the AIDS Crisis* was published, and the first conference on women and AIDS, organized jointly by Pandora Press and the Terrence Higgins Trust, was held in London in May of that year. A handful of short articles by feminist writers also appeared, in response to growing awareness of both the disease itself and its implications for women. Interestingly, given the usual association of sexuality with a radical feminist agenda, these included articles by socialist feminist writers such as Beatrix Campbell (in *Marxism Today*) and Lynne Segal (in *New Socialist*). (Also, see Segal's later piece on feminism and AIDS (1989) and Segal (1990).) *Spare Rib* in its April and May issues ran features on women and AIDS, and in the summer of 1987 the radical feminist magazine *Trouble and Strife* published an article which looked explicitly at the lack of feminist contribution to debates about AIDS (Scott, 1987). The British socialist feminist journal *Feminist Review* first addressed the issue of AIDS a year later, in 1988, with an article by American AIDS activist Cindy Patton on 'Lessons from the Gay Community'.

Since then, there has been a steady (if not vast) output of work by feminist writers reflecting the diversity of issues surrounding women and AIDS. This includes, for instance, books by Ines Rieder and Patricia Ruppelt (1988) *AIDS: The Women,* the Panos Institute (1990) *Triple Jeopardy: Women and AIDS,* the ACT UP/New York Women and AIDS Book Group (1990) *Women, AIDS and Activism,* Diane Richardson (1990a) *Safer Sex: The Guide for Women Today,* the Women, Risk and AIDS Project (WRAP) papers (for example, Holland *et al.,* 1990), Sue O'Sullivan and Kate Thomson (1992) *Positively*

Women: Living with AIDS, Judy Bury, Val Morrison and Sheena McLachlan (1992) *Working with Women and AIDS,* Marge Berer with Sunanda Ray (1993) *Women and HIV/AIDS: An International Resource Book,* and Corinne Squire (1993) *Women and AIDS: Psychological Perspectives.* Articles about women and AIDS have also occasionally appeared in *Spare Rib, Feminist Review* (issues 34 (1990) and 41 (1992)) and *Trouble and Strife* (Cameron, 1992).

The literature representing lesbian feminist thought on AIDS has been even more limited. There has been work published on the various issues HIV/AIDS raises for lesbians, including the question of woman-to-woman transmission (e.g. Patton and Kelly, 1987; Leonard, 1990). Also, the British journal of lesbian feminist ethics, *Gossip,* published a number of articles and letters on AIDS, including Vada Hart's (1986) controversial early piece which stated that AIDS is not an issue for lesbians and declared that 'LESBIAN SEX IS SAFE'. This is a view which has been encouraged by the failure of most researchers and health educators to address lesbians in discussions of women and AIDS. A few writers, however, have included in their work discussion about why and how lesbians might want to adopt safer sex practices (e.g. Richardson, 1987; Patton, 1990; O'Sullivan and Parmar, 1993), including, in 1987, an article in the British gay magazine *Square Peg* outlining safer sex guidelines for lesbians. (Interestingly, the Terrence Higgins Trust did not produce an information leaflet about HIV and AIDS for lesbians until October, 1990.)

On a political level, some writers have acknowledged how the potential for AIDS to challenge traditional beliefs about sexuality could have positive implications for lesbians (e.g. Ardill and O'Sullivan, 1987; Campbell, 1987; Richardson, 1989). The disagreement and divisions between lesbian feminists over the political relevance of HIV/AIDS for lesbians has also been written about (see, for instance, Boffin, 1990; Cameron, 1992). There are some lesbian feminists who feel that lesbians should avoid campaigning and organizing around HIV/AIDS, because it marginalizes and draws energy away from lesbian/feminist concerns (e.g. Hart, 1986). Nevertheless, many lesbian/feminists, both in the United States and in Europe, are involved in HIV/AIDS work and are AIDS activists. Accounts by lesbians involved in AIDS politics of some of the difficulties and contradictions they may face are provided in, for example, Rieder and Ruppelt (1989), Schneider (1992), Smyth (1992) and Winnow (1992).

The main themes to emerge from this small body of feminist work on women and HIV/AIDS are: implications of HIV/AIDS for women as a health issue: the importance for feminism of public debates on HIV/AIDS; reproductive rights issues raised by HIV/AIDS; racism, women and HIV/AIDS; the representation of women in the HIV/AIDS discourse; notions of safer sex and the problems for women of negotiating sex on their terms; evaluation of health education aimed at women; the impact of HIV/AIDS on specific groups of women such as carers of people with HIV-related disease, injecting drug users, lesbians, and women who work as prostitutes; the experience of women who are HIV-positive, have AIDS and/or are working around these issues; and, finally, the relationship between AIDS politics and feminism.

AIDS Is a Feminist Issue

It is one thing to say that AIDS is a women's issue, another to claim that it is a feminist issue. The latter demands that we ask not only how HIV/ AIDS affects women specifically, but also how women's subordination influences their risk status and experience of HIV/AIDS. In what ways does the unequal position of women in society play a significant role in HIV infection in women? There is also the question of the extent to which women's ability to reduce their risk of infection, and the impact that HIV/AIDS has on their lives, is not merely a reflection of their unequal position in society, but also reinforces male power and control over women. Do HIV/AIDS or, more specifically, social and political responses to HIV/AIDS actually increase women's oppression?

Whilst a number of contributions to the literature on women and AIDS are informed by feminist theory, there has to date been very little written from a specifically feminist standpoint. Few writers have moved beyond acknowledging gender differences and outlining the specific ways in which HIV/AIDS affects women differently to men such as, for example, in the process of negotiating safer sex and the gender-specific issue of transmission of HIV during pregnancy and the process of birth. That there has been little analysis of the above questions is all the more striking when one considers the issues raised by HIV/AIDS. Many of these — such as control over sexuality, reproductive freedom, women's access to health care — are old issues for feminism, about which feminists have campaigned long and hard. As Sara Scott (1987) comments:

> AIDS has created the biggest public debate on sexuality, sexual practice and sexual morality since the media recovered from the shock of the 'sixties; yet it is one to which feminists have yet to make a particular contribution. Our silence seems bizarre

because the issues raised by AIDS are very much on our political patch. (Scott, 1987, p. 13)

What are some of the possible reasons for this?

Why Have Feminists Failed to Involve Themselves in the AIDS Debate?

'AIDS Isn't a Women's Issue'

Looking back over the 1980s it is clear that much of what has been said or written about AIDS has been coloured by an overwhelming, if unstated, assumption that AIDS is a disease of men (Panos, 1990). From the beginning, in the West, AIDS was identified as a white gay men's problem. The media played a significant role in constructing this view, frequently referring to AIDS as the 'gay disease' or the 'gay plague'. This, coupled with a dearth of information and lack of discussion about women and AIDS, may explain why at first many feminists did not identify AIDS as a 'women's issue' (even though lesbians, subsumed under the category homosexual, were often perceived as 'high-risk'!). The relatively small number of women diagnosed with AIDS in Britain (61 as of October 1988, compared to 1,801 men) may also have contributed to the initial lack of feminist activism around AIDS. There is another possible reason for this, besides women's invisibility. Speaking about the situation in Victoria, Australia, Anne Mitchell (1992) claims that when the number of women infected with HIV is low, these women not only suffer from marginalization and a lack of appropriate services:

they are also a group rightly fearful for their privacy and an inevitable backlash against themselves and their children. Personal activism or energetic attempts to excite the ire of feminist advocates to act on their behalf can therefore be seen as threatening and out of the question. (Mitchell, 1992, p. 52)

The fact that AIDS politics was initially (and many would argue still is) dominated by gay men also tended to confirm the lack of political relevance for women. For this reason some would ask whether it is politically desirable for feminists to put their energies into AIDS work and activism. This is a view which, I think, is shared by many feminists.

They can see that HIV and AIDS affect women in specific ways that are politically significant, but equally feel that such issues are likely to be marginalized in AIDS politics — so why bother? The attempt by some gay men to 're-gay' AIDS, as part of an understandable response to the way that gay men have become more and more invisible in the provision of government-funded education and services around HIV and AIDS, has sometimes fuelled this view and led to disagreement and divisions between gay men and women asserting their respective need of AIDS resources.

> some gay men are now claiming that lesbians working in HIV and AIDS are taking up valuable resources at a point where gay men continue to be the main group affected in Britain and other northern European countries. Within this scenario, lesbians are criticized simply for pointing out the lack of knowledge about women and HIV. (O'Sullivan and Parmar, 1993, pp. 23–4).

Whilst the possible marginalization of the needs of women in relation to HIV and AIDS is an understandable concern, the argument that we should therefore not get involved in AIDS politics is short-sighted. What it demonstrates is the need for a clearer feminist agenda on HIV/AIDS which, although it would undoubtably be influenced by the politics of AIDS, would prioritize a feminist politics in particular of sexuality and health. Some feminists would still question whether it is politically desirable to make alliances with gay men, although clearly others would disagree as is evident with the emergence of mixed activist groups like ACT UP, OutRage and Queer Nation.

'We've Got Enough on our Plate Already without AIDS'

At present, in the West, there are many more deaths in women as a result of breast cancer (and cervical cancer) than are caused by HIV-related disease. This, and the fact that there is no provision for research and prevention on a similar scale to HIV and AIDS, is perhaps why some feminists in the women's health movement have seen HIV/AIDS as of minor importance, relative to wider health issues for women.

Another explanation for the lack of feminist involvement in AIDS politics is that AIDS is perceived as a low priority issue for feminism generally in the nineties. This begs the question, of course, of why this should be the case given that HIV and AIDS raises issues that feminists are familiar with. Is it merely the case that we do not recognize the issues in the context of HIV and AIDS or, more fundamentally, does it reflect the importance (or lack of it) placed on these issues within contemporary feminist theory and debate? AIDS demands that we develop feminist critiques of heterosexuality as well as of the politics of the feminist health movement, issues that dominated feminist debates in the seventies. However, times change, and for many feminists women's health issues and feminist analyses of compulsory heterosexuality are no longer of central concern (Cameron, 1992).

AIDS raises old issues for feminism and maybe that is just it: is lack of interest the result of a kind of political ageism that celebrates the 'new'? There is also another way of looking at this. Because many of the issues AIDS raises are ones that feminists have been tackling for a very long time it has less immediate impact; holds fewer suprises; is in many ways a confirmation of past feminist concerns rather than a challenge to them. Arguably, AIDS lacks the power to repoliticize feminism in the way it has gay politics. In this sense, feminist lack of attention to AIDS and HIV specifically could be seen, in part, as the outcome of assimilation to a broader political agenda, and not simply as a political stratagem or a fashion in feminist thinking.

'All that AIDS stuff — it pisses me off'

It is also important to recognize that many feminists feel angered by the attention given to HIV and AIDS when other serious health issues that women face, such as breast cancer, have never received the same level of funding or interest (Winnow, 1992). They may also feel angry because feminists raising similar issues in a different context have been ignored. Both earlier this century and more recently, feminists have been concerned with 'safer sex', in particular the prevention of unwanted pregnancy, health risks associated with contraceptive use and sexual abuse. It is therefore somewhat galling to observe the ways in which the government, media and medical profession have responded to the 'AIDS crisis'. Why this attention to 'safer sex' now? 'It seems as if only now, when men's health is at stake, do we need to consider sexual risks and responsibilities' (Richardson, 1990b, p. 175).

Similarly, Ros Coward, commenting on HIV/AIDS public education campaigns, remarks:

> There are some especially cruel ironies for feminism in the current situation. We have to watch general pressure mounting to transform sexual innuendo in advertising yet feminist

campaigns against sexism in adverts have largely failed. Especially cruel is the conclusion of the British Government AIDS leaflet: 'Ultimately, defence against the disease depends on all of us taking responsibility for our own actions'. The feminist call for men to do just that has been something of a voice in the wilderness in the past'. (Coward, 1987, p. 21)

It is partly for these reasons that many feminists have contradictory responses to AIDS, which may influence their willingness to get involved in HIV/AIDS work and debates.

What Are the Implications of a Lack of Feminist Input?

In the AIDS crisis, women are most of the time completely invisible, face severe and sometimes insurmountable obstacles to coming out with a positive HIV status, are rarely provided with adequate care, and have to take care of the most people. (The ACT UP/New York Women and AIDS Book Group, 1990, p. 243).

Whatever the reasons for the muted response of feminism to HIV/AIDS, to date, it is clear that this has important implications for policy-making, particularly in relation to women who are HIV-positive or have AIDS. The view of men as 'the norm' in the AIDS crisis has not only helped to render women invisible to researchers and those involved in the diagnosis and treatment of HIV and AIDS, it has also shaped the development of, for example, educational, housing, health and social services policies. Consequently, it is not surprising to find that many such policies do not successfully meet women's specific needs.

Such a situation cries out for a feminist response not only in challenging assumptions of policy-makers, but also in providing a theoretical framework for understanding women's position in the AIDS crisis — which could inform the policy-making process and help determine service provision. AIDS education policies are unlikely to be effective unless they acknowledge male control over women's sexuality and reproductive capacities. The development of health and social services to care for and support people with AIDS or other HIV-related illness, and those looking after them, demands an understanding of women's unpaid work in the home, in particular their responsibility for the care of family members. Housing policies need to recognize both women's position in the labour market and the fact that they bear disproportionate responsibility for childcare. It is, in part, failure to address these issues which has so far prevented women from receiving adequate information and services. In outlining a feminist agenda on HIV/AIDS, therefore, we need to respond to these issues, not least by drawing attention also to the way HIV/AIDS service providers may have a lot to learn from feminist health movements.

Other feminist writers are more directly concerned that AIDS has become a major focus for public debates about sexuality and sexual politics, and that by not being a part of this discourse we are not only failing to contribute to an understanding of issues which concern us politically, we are also missing the boat. Ros Coward (1987), for instance, argues for greater feminist engagement in discussions about AIDS partly because she thinks it would be 'foolish and defeatist' not to do so, but also because she sees AIDS as an opportunity to redefine sexuality and negotiate new meanings. AIDS potentially challenges what is considered 'natural' or 'normal' about sexuality, in particular the focus on sex as penetration. More fundamentally, AIDS provides an opportunity to discuss the balance of power between women and men, and the role sexuality plays in the maintenance of men's power over women. Other feminist writers (e.g. Holland *et al.*, 1990; Richardson, 1989) have acknowledged this in their work. Sara Scott (1987), for instance, has this to say:

> Ironically, AIDS has promoted the open discussion of sexual practice on an unprecedented scale. We should seize the opportunity to get into the debate, proposing alternatives to a penetrative heterosexual morality and place a radical, feminist analysis of sexuality firmly on the agenda. (Scott, 1987, p. 18)

If feminism has, so far, failed to take up the challenges which AIDS poses, then it is also the case that much of the HIV/AIDS discourse has so far failed to acknowledge and/or incorporate feminist theory and research about sexuality. In particular, health education policy and the medical establishment have tended to ignore what feminists have had to say about the role of sexuality in women's lives. Within feminist theory sexuality is identified as a site of struggle in which men exercise power over women, although important differences exist between feminists in the significance attributed to sexuality in understanding women's oppression. Acknowledging the power relations embedded in sexual relations helps to explain both how and why women can find the process of negotiating safer sex difficult. As Janet Holland *et al.*, point out:

> From a feminist perspective, using or not using a condom is not a simple, practical question about dealing rationally with risk, it is the outcome of negotiation between potentially unequal partners. ... In many sexual encounters women have little choice about whether or how to engage in sexual activity with men, the options being physical injury or more subtle forms of sanction. (Holland, *et al.*, 1990, p. 5)

Most public education campaigns around AIDS and HIV, in assuming individual choice and personal responsibility, do not address the issue of relative power in sexual relations. This not only limits how effective such campaigns are likely to be, it also relegates women's difficulties in translating knowledge into practice to the level of individual excuses. This has potentially important implications for blame, especially given the tendency within debates about heterosexual transmission to focus on women as primarily responsible for HIV prevention. For example, in March 1989 the Health Education Authority (HEA) launched their first major advertising campaign targeted at women, with the aim of encouraging women to ask their male partners to use a condom. Unfortunately, what the HEA did not do was run a parallel campaign directed at heterosexual men. They thus reinforced the belief that it is women who are primarily responsible for safer sex and, by implication, heterosexual transmission of HIV. (Since then the Health Education Authority has made some attempts to specifically target heterosexual men as well as women, for instance in the television campaign it ran in 1992.)

In addition to the lack of acknowledgment of sexual inequalities, feminist work has been ignored in other ways. To listen to what many have to say about AIDS you would think sex had never before been dangerous, as if sex pre-AIDS were all hearts and flowers, fun and games, a time of splendour when we all could be spontaneous and do whatever we wanted to sexually without worrying about the possible risks to ourselves or our partners. It is as if feminists had never criticized sexual relationships between men and women, with the emphasis on vaginal intercourse as, very often, unsatisfying and/or dangerous for women. Many nineteenth-century feminists drew attention to the ways in which sex was dangerous to women, in particular through the debilitating effect of repeated pregnancies and infection from venereal diseases such as syphilis (see Jeffreys, 1985). More recently, in the early 1970s, many feminists voiced criticisms of heterosexuality as a form of sexual practice (e.g. Koedt, 1974). In particular, they challenged the centrality of sexual intercourse in heterosexual relations, pointing out that very often this is not the major or only source of sexual arousal for women. Such debates were important in acknowledging the many ways of obtaining sexual pleasure through non-penetrative means. In other words, feminists have had a great deal to say about 'safer sex', yet this has been virtually ignored.

One of the consequences of this has been the construction of a concept of safer sex which, in largely ignoring feminist analyses of sexuality, has marginalized more traditional feminist concerns about sexual practice. As Deborah Cameron (1992) points out:

> The whole question of what constitutes 'safe sex' has come to be defined in terms of whether a particular sexual practice is more or less likely to transmit HIV: the sense in which pornography and phone sex might actually threaten the physical or psychological safety of women, or be open to criticism on other grounds, is glossed over in this discourse where safer sex is better and 'safer' means 'carrying lower HIV risk'. (Cameron, 1992, p. 44)

This is something which has rarely been addressed in feminist contributions to the HIV/AIDS discourse. What discussion there has been has tended to focus mainly on the way in which — ironically, given what we know about HIV transmission — much of the safer sex discourse reaffirms rather than challenges the notion of 'sex' as vaginal intercourse (e.g. Campbell, 1987; Scott, 1987). In most AIDS prevention efforts the emphasis is on having fewer sexual partners and the correct use of condoms as the best way of making sex 'safe'. There is very little discussion of non-penetrative sex, and what there is often appears apologetic.

Some have also critized the way in which safer sex is defined for other reasons, drawing attention to the problematic nature of discussing safer sex primarily in terms of sexual practices which are more or less likely to transmit HIV. From a feminist perspective the concept of 'safer sex' incorporates much broader concerns.

> It (safer sex) is also about not getting other sexually transmitted diseases, making sure you don't become pregnant unless you want to be, reducing the health risks associated with certain forms of contraception and preventing cervical cancer. We can also think about safer sex in another way. There are all sorts of

reasons why sex for women is often unsafe for emotional as well as physical reasons. Women get raped and sexually abused. Women often feel pressurized into having sex just to please their partner . . . When we feel forced into having sex it can shatter our self-esteem. It can leave us feeling exploited and used. Safer sex is about sex we enjoy and feel good about. It's about sex on our terms; sex that reduces the risks to our minds as well as our bodies! (Richardson, 1990a, pp. 34–5).

From this perspective, it is possible to critique the promotion of certain practices as 'safer sex' *despite* their involving little or no risk of transmission of HIV. Take, for example, the suggestion that sharing sexual fantasies is safe. Whilst this may be true in terms of the prevention of sexually transmitted disease and unwanted pregnancy, from a feminist perspective there are other potential risks to consider. Fantasies which conflict with our feelings and values can be, ultimately, psychologically unsafe. Similarly, if fantasy be the stuff of safer sex, then it is easy to see how this can be used to defend pornography. Tamsin Wilton (this volume) highlights the difficulties of regarding pornography as safe sex.

How Does AIDS Inform Feminist Theory and Practice?

In addition to considering the implications of a lack of feminist theorizing on how we understand and respond to HIV and AIDS, we also need to ask what the implications for feminist theory and practice of the HIV/AIDS epidemic are. As I have suggested earlier, at one level AIDS has reminded us (in case we needed reminding) that sexuality is still a central concern. Research on how women are at risk, and how they can best protect themselves, highlights how men's power over women, economically and socially, affects sexual relationships and constrains women's options for HIV prevention, as well as for safer sex more generally. Furthermore, AIDS not only highlights the potential dangers of heterosexuality as a form of sexual practice, it also underlines the importance of heterosexuality as a primary institution of women's oppression. This can be evidenced in a number of ways, for example in the way that women outside of 'normal' married, heterosexual relations have often been represented within the AIDS discourse. Lesbians, bisexual women, women who work as prostitutes and sexually active single women have all, to varying extents, been deemed responsible for the spread of AIDS. It is also evident in the concern to situate sexuality within a reproductive, marital context, especially for women.

Another example is the way in which AIDS has impacted on women's lives as carers of people with HIV/AIDS. Here the issue is women's traditional role as unpaid caregiver within the heterosexual family and the negative consequences this can often have for women's own health and the services they receive. Motherhood is an important aspect of the institution of heterosexuality, and here again many of the reproductive rights issues connected with HIV and AIDS, such as the routine testing of pregnant women for HIV antibodies and the carrying out of forced abortions and compulsory sterilizations on HIV-positive women, are attempts at preventing the spread of AIDS through the control of women's fertility. As Jalna Hanmer (1993) has pointed out, the focus on the control of women's fertility through contraception, abortion or sterilization masks the issue of men's assumed 'right' of sexual access to women.

In addition to the issue of women's relative lack of control over sexuality and reproductive capacities, HIV/AIDS raises many other issues, such as access to health care, housing and childcare facilities, which are long-term goals of feminism. HIV/AIDS has also, once again, highlighted the low priority given to research about women's health needs. Having said this, it is important to consider how feminist theory and practice, as well as being validated in certain respects, might need to be modified in the light of our understanding of HIV/AIDS and how it influences women's lives in varying ways. For instance, feminist services such as women's refuges and rape crisis centres now need to incorporate into their work the issues of women being battered for demanding safer sex and the worry of HIV infection as part of the trauma of having been raped. Other services such as lesbian telephone helplines are also having to adapt their practices in the light of HIV/AIDS issues.

At another level, we need to consider the impact of HIV/AIDS on prevailing ideologies of sexuality and ask how this may, for example, alter the meanings associated with lesbianism and heterosexuality, as well as how we theorize these sexualities. AIDS has revitalized a conservative sexual politics which seeks to strengthen traditional, heterosexual family values and associate homosexuality and sex outside of marriage with sin and disease. We must ask what effect this is likely to have on the construction of sexual subjectivities (especially non-heterosexual ones) and on male control within marriage.

At the same time, we need to recognize that AIDS has also become the symbol for a very different kind of sexual politics. It represents, for some, the symbol of a 'progressive' sexual politics; one that according to Lynne Segal (1990) is at 'the cutting edge of sexual politics today'. This is a politics of 'radical pluralism' (if not sexual libertarianism) which has grown out of divisions within feminism as well as AIDS activism; a politics which has also emerged, at least in part, in response to the conservatism that has been revitalized by AIDS. The question is, how far does it relate to feminist politics of sexuality?

For some feminists it clearly does. The 1980s saw a number of splits within feminism over issues like pornography and lesbian sadomasochism, and the emergence of so-called 'pro-sex', anti-censorship feminists, some of whom have been attracted to mixed organizations like ACT UP and a (postmodern?) politics of sexuality which affirms individual sexual choice and the diversity of sexual desire. Cherry Smyth (1992), for example, implies that this new queer politics liberates sexual theory (and practice) from the restrictions of a 'prescriptive feminism'. Similarly, the writer Sarah Shulman, quoted in Smyth (1992), claims that: 'AIDS activism is far more effective than feminism ever was because it allows a broad diversity of opinion, while in feminism there was a tendency to block a range of analysis'.

Others take a very different view and are concerned that the libertarian influence within AIDS politics has resulted in an insufficient critique of the relationship between sexuality and power and, related to this, the notions of individual choice and consent.

> A *feminist* politics of sexuality must surely give weight to both choice and compulsion as dimensions of women's experience around sex. The right to say yes and the power to say no are both important. AIDS politics, dominated initially by gay men, have tended to be about affirming sexual choice . . . (Cameron, 1992, p. 45)

Some would go further in arguing that much of the radical political work on HIV/AIDS is not merely insufficient in its treatment of sexuality and gender (and 'race'), it is specifically anti-feminist (Wilton, 1992). Certainly, as I have indicated above, there is a very real concern that the focus on HIV and AIDS in current debates about sexuality may lead to the marginalization of traditional feminist concerns about sexuality. What it also does — ironically — is underline the importance of heterosexuality as a central concern for feminism in the nineties.

References

THE ACT UP/NEW YORK WOMEN AND AIDS BOOK GROUP (1990) *Women, AIDS and Activism,* Boston, South End Press.

ARDILL, SUSAN and O'SULLIVAN, SUE (1987) 'AIDS and Women: Building a Feminist Framework', *Spare Rib*, May.

BERER, MARGE with RAY, SUNANDA (1993) *Women and HIV/AIDS: An International Resource Book*, London, Pandora Press.

BOFFIN, TESSA (1990) 'Fairy Tales, "Facts" And Gossip: Lesbians and AIDS', in BOFFIN, TESSA and GUPTA, SUNIL (Eds) *Ecstatic Antibodies: Resisting the AIDS Mythology*, London, Rivers Oram Press.

BURY, JUDY, MORRISON, VAL and MCLACHLAN, SHEENA (Eds) (1992) *Working with Women and AIDS: Medical, Social and Counselling Issues*, London, Routledge.

CAMERON, DEBORAH (1992) 'Old Het?', *Trouble and Strife*, no. 24.

CAMPBELL, BEATRIX (1987) 'Taking the Plunge', *Marxism Today*, December, p. 9.

COWARD, ROS (1987) 'Sex after AIDS', *New Internationalist*, March, pp. 20-1.

HANMER, JALNA (1993) 'Women and Reproduction', in RICHARDSON, DIANE and ROBINSON, VICTORIA, (Eds) *Introducing Women's Studies: Feminist Theory and Practice*, London, Macmillan.

HART, VADA (1986) 'Lesbians and A.I.D.S.', *Gossip: A Journal of Lesbian Feminist Ethics*, no. 2.

HOLLAND, JANET, RAMAZANOGLU, CAROLINE, SCOTT, SUE, SHARPE, SUE and THOMSON, RACHEL (1990) '"Don't Die of Ignorance — I Nearly Died of Embarrassment": Condoms in Context', WRAP Paper 2, London, Tufnell Press.

JEFFREYS, SHEILA (1985) *The Spinster and Her Enemies: Feminism and Sexuality 1880-1930*, London, Pandora Press.

KAPLAN, HELEN SINGER (1987) *The Real Truth About Women and AIDS: How to Eliminate the Risks Without Giving Up Love and Sex*, New York, Simon and Schuster.

KOEDT, ANNE (1974) 'The Myth of the Vaginal Orgasm'. In The Radical Therapist Collective (Eds), *The Radical Therapist*, Harmondsworth, Penguin.

LEONARD, ZOE (1990) 'Lesbians in the AIDS Crisis', in THE ACT UP/NEW YORK WOMEN AND AIDS BOOK GROUP *Women, AIDS and Activism*, Boston, South End Press.

MITCHELL, ANNE (1992) 'Women and AIDS Activism in Victoria, Australia', *Feminist Review*, no. 41, pp. 52-7.

NORWOOD, CHRIS (1987) *Advice for Life: A Woman's Guide to AIDS Risks and Prevention*, New York, Pantheon Books.

O'SULLIVAN, SUE and PARMAR, PRATIBHA (1993) *Lesbians Talk (Safer) Sex*, London, Scarlet Press.

O'SULLIVAN, SUE and THOMSON, KATE (Eds) (1992) *Positively Women: Living with AIDS*, London, Sheba.

PANOS INSTITUTE (1990) *Triple Jeopardy: Women and AIDS*, London, The Panos Institute.

PATTON, CINDY (1988) 'AIDS: Lessons from the Gay Community', *Feminist Review*, no. 30, pp. 105-11.

PATTON, CINDY (1990), 'Mapping: Lesbianism, AIDS and Sexuality', *Feminist Review*, 34, pp. 120-33.

PATTON, CINDY and KELLY, JANIS (1987) *Making It: A Woman's Guide to Sex in the Age of AIDS*, Ithaca, New York, Firebrand Books.

RICHARDSON, DIANE (1987/1989) *Women and the AIDS Crisis*, London, Pandora Press (2nd edition, 1989).

RICHARDSON, DIANE (1990a) *Safer Sex: The Guide for Women Today*, London, Pandora Press.

RICHARDSON, DIANE (1990b) 'AIDS Education and Women: Sexual and Reproductive Issues', in AGGLETON, PETER, DAVIES, PETER and HART, GRAHAM (Eds) *AIDS: Individual, Cultural and Policy Dimensions*, London, Falmer Press.

RIEDER, INES and RUPPELT, PATRICIA (Eds) (1988) *AIDS: The Women*,

RIEDER, INES and RUPPELT, PATRICIA (Eds) (1989) *Matters of Life and Death: Women Speak about AIDS,* London, Virago.

RUDD, ANDREA and TAYLOR, DARIEN (Eds) (1992) *Positive Women: Voices of Women Living with AIDS,* Toronto, Second Story Press.

SCHNEIDER, BETH E. (1992) 'Lesbian Politics and AIDS Work', in PLUMMBER, KEN (Ed.) *Modern Homosexualities,* London, Routledge.

SCOTT, SARA (1987) 'Sex and Danger: Feminism and AIDS', *Trouble and Strife,* no. 11.

SEGAL, LYNNE (1987) 'AIDS is a Feminist Issue', *New Socialist,* April.

SEGAL, LYNNE (1989) 'Lessons from the Past: Feminism, Sexual Politics and the Challenge of AIDS', in CARTER, ERICA and WATNEY, SIMON (Eds) *Taking Liberties: AIDS and Cultural Politics,* London, Serpent's Tail.

SEGAL, LYNNE (1990) *Slow Motion: Changing Masculinities, Changing Men,* London, Virago.

SMYTH, CHERRY (1992) *Lesbians Talk Queer Notions,* London, Scarlet Press.

SQUIRE, CORINNE (Ed.) (1993) *Women and AIDS: Psychological Perspectives,* London, Sage.

WILTON, TAMSIN (1992) 'Desire and the Politics of Representation: Issues for Lesbians and Heterosexual Women', in HINDS, HILARY, PHOENIX, ANN and STACEY, JACKIE (Eds) *Working Out: New Directions for Women's Studies,* London, Falmer Press.

WINNOW, JACKIE (1992) 'Lesbians Evolving Health Care: Cancer and AIDS', *Feminist Review,* no. 41, pp. 68–76.

Section II

The Disputed Body

Chapter 4

Desire, Risk and Control:
The Body as a Site of Contestation

Janet Holland, Caroline Ramazanoglu, Sue Scott and Rachel Thomson

Introduction

After a long period of neglect, the body is emerging as a legitimate focus and locus of social science enquiry (Turner, 1984; Featherstone *et al.*, 1991; Scott and Morgan, 1992). With this surge of theorizing, battleground metaphors have come to the fore and power struggles are seen as being played out on the field of the body. The nature of the battles being fought, however, and the meaning of the body as a contested site are far from agreed. Most of the academic discussion of the body has taken place in debates between philosophers or at a level of considerable abstraction, so that those not versed in poststructuralism, postmodernism and critiques of Cartesian dualisms can be left floundering.[1]

Yet our bodies are at some level the basis of our material existence — our few pleasures and our many pains. If women are to confront the global AIDS epidemic with effective strategies for safer sex, then we need to understand, recognize and so control and take care of our own bodies. Although the safest sex is practised alone, sex as a social activity means negotiating sexual practices with partners. If heterosexual women are to be able to control their bodies, they must come to terms with the ways in which the social construction of masculinity and femininity estranges women from their bodies.[2] The relation of the 'properly' feminine body to women is not the same as the relation of the 'properly' masculine body to men. Safeguarding our bodies means being able to assert and express women's desires as well as men's and, therefore, being able to understand and respond to the risks we run in heterosexual encounters. Safer sex requires that women embody their own desires; that they are informed about their bodies and the risks they can run; that they know about the possiblities of desires and passions, recognize what these feel like, and are able to value them. This kind of embodiment provides a social space within which women and men can negotiate sexual encounters so as to ensure that sexual safety is a shared concern. Sexual safety cannot, however, develop in isolation in the privacy of sexual encounters, since these encounters are constrained by the more general institutionalization of gendered power relations.

In this chapter, we consider what a feminist understanding of the body could mean with reference to strategies for safer sex. We look briefly at the tension between the approaches to the body which have been taken by feminists and by Foucault. This general topic is grounded in a specific study of 150 young women in London and Manchester, UK, who were interviewed between 1988 and 1990 about the ways in which they negotiated sexual encounters with men.[3] Drawing on these data we explore the ways in which young women understand and experience their bodies and their sexuality, illustrating the power struggles played out in this field through an examination of their knowledge of sexuality, and issues raised by their accounts of desire, risk and control. We argue that the young women's limited sexual knowledge, their alienation from their own desires, and the concomitant lack of control in sexual encounters places them at particular risk in relation to HIV infection.

The Disputed Body: Feminism versus Foucault

Moira Gatens (1988) has pointed out that feminists have made women's bodies a focal point around which struggles for autonomy have been fought. Conflict around women's rights to contraception, abortion, control of childbirth and pleasure have clearly been central to feminism. In battles for control of the body, men in general have been seen as having power over women, and therefore as ranged politically against women. This view of gendered power which is so central to feminism is, however, disputed by Foucault and his poststructuralist followers. Feminist theory has developed with little reference to his theory of the body, sexuality and the nature of power, while Foucault has largely ignored feminism. Analysis of the tensions between Foucault and feminism can be a productive way of understanding the disembodiment of femininity, and so the problems of achieving safer sex.

Radical feminists have long argued that the material basis of women's oppression is located in men's control of women's bodies, with male power exercised through men's control over female sexuality and reproductive capacity. At an abstract level, the concept of patriarchy has helped to conceptualize the nature of male power; at a more empirical level, feminist studies have conceptualized and documented the ways in which the exercise and threat of male violence is entwined with sexuality. Women's ability to control and safeguard their bodies opposes female autonomy to patriarchal power, but feminist theory of the body is relatively underdeveloped. This underdevelopment of theory of the body is linked to the underdevelopment of a feminist theory of power (Hartsock, 1983).

Foucault's ideas on power and the body offer a potential critique of feminism. Foucault argues that we need a history of feelings, behaviour and the body (Foucault, 1988, p. 112). Rather than describing our present sexual misery (*ibid.*, p. 113) we need to grasp the positive mechanisms which produce sexuality in this or that fashion. This view can be taken as identifying a trap of implicit biological essentialism in feminism, even where this is not intended (Dworkin, 1988), in which the body is taken to be biologically fixed.

In our interpretations of the accounts of their sexual encounters given by young women, we intend to avoid this trap by taking the biological and the social to be inextricably entwined. 'Biology provides a *bedrock* for social inscription but is not a fixed or static substratum: it interacts with and is overlaid by psychic, social and signifying relations' (Grosz, 1990, p. 72). The material body and its desires are given meaning through processes of social construction; ideas about the body are social, but are not entirely separable from bodily constraints and possibilities.[4]

Foucault's work also raises problems for feminist conceptions of patriarchy and women's liberation. In his view we cannot understand power as a possession which can be held by a group or groups in society. As there is no such possession, then there cannot be patriarchal power held by men and opposed by women. According to Foucault, power is diffuse rather than located in some central group, institution or source. Gender then cannot be a source of power. This does not mean that power is shared. Some categories of people will be subjected to power exercised by others, and their bodies will be disciplined and controlled (for example, in schools, prisons, hospitals). But in this view there can be no monolithic patriarchal power; it has to be plural, precarious and unstable. Power is exercised through a shifting constellation of discourses, techniques and practices.[5]

Foucault (1980a, p. 186) attempts to 'show how power relations can materially penetrate the body in depth, without depending even on the mediation of the subject's own representation'. For Foucault, the body is changeable, since it is a social site in which ideas and discourses about sexuality are played out. This view has been developed in isolation from feminist work on gendered power, but is not incompatible with it in all respects. Our data support the view that sexuality is a field in which detailed techniques of power are exercised on the body. The body is both material and, at the same time, a social space where the larger-scale organization of power is connected to minute and local practices (Sawicki, 1991). The study of strategies for achieving safer sex can benefit from considering Foucault's understanding of power, but feminists remain critical of Foucault in retaining the conception of gendered power.

Foucault emphasizes that the body is both a target of power, since it is constituted by discourses (for example by current medical knowledge or approved models of sex education) and also site of resistance. The meaning of resistance is one point where feminist politics diverge from Foucault's relativism and pluralism (Hekman, 1990). From a feminist perspective, Foucault's theory is flawed because he simply followed in an established male-centred, philosophical tradition (which he perhaps recognized, but did not really respond to) by ignoring both feminist work and also the specificity of women's experience (Morris, 1979; Schor, 1987). He does not allow for the ways in which women experience gendered power.

Braidotti (1991, p. 96) summarizes the problems of Foucault's position by arguing that he is trapped in a gender-blind theoretical discourse, which is not just politically unacceptable but, in leaving women out, is inaccurate as theory: 'the notion of power which Foucault develops rests on a masculine view of the body'. Although he identifies the body as a site of power, he rejects the idea of women confronting a patriarchal system.

> The real strength of the women's liberation movements is not that of having laid claim to the specificity of their sexuality and the rights pertaining to it, but that they have actually departed from the discourse conducted within the apparatuses of sexuality. (Foucault, 1980b, pp. 219–20).

Women in his view can dismantle the categories of masculine and feminine by creating new discourses of sexuality. He does not conceive of women as needing to liberate their material bodies from gendered power. Men's power over women, and the strength of men's daily (and often violent) control of women's bodies is not conceptualized in this perspective (Holland *et al.*, 1992c). Other links between, for example, slavery, racism and the social construction of gender are also not recognized.[6]

This confrontation between feminism and Foucault can be a

positive one for understanding the problems of achieving safer sex if feminists consider the problems of thinking about power which Foucault raises (Barrett, 1991; Bartky, 1990; Hekman, 1990). His criticism that too much has been assumed about power *structures* and that not enough attention has been paid to exactly *how* power is exercised and contested is useful (Foucault, 1988, p. 103). Analysis of the problems faced by young women in trying to control and care for their bodies indicates that they both support and resist gendered power.

The question of what it means for women to resist men's power over their material bodies is examined here in terms of what it means for young women to be able to control and take care of their own bodies. Safer sex is not a matter of rational decision-making between equal agents, but a complex and unstable process of negotiation between gendered beings where not only is the masculine socially privileged over the feminine, but female heterosexuality is socially constructed to support male dominance. The extent of male privilege in sexual encounters is clarified in the next section through consideration of what constitutes young women's sexual knowledge, and what is expressed by them as desire.

Sexual Knowledge and the Silencing of Desire

Young women's understandings of their bodies are shaped and constrained by the processes of social construction of gender which provide limited ways in which they can recognize and legitimate their bodily experiences and practices. Women are not simply passively conditioned to accept socially dominant ideas, rules and values. If they are to be able to resist constructions of femininity in which they contribute to their own subordination, however, they have to have both a critical consciousness of disembodied femininity and effective strategies for their own empowerment (Holland *et al.*, 1992a). The ways in which young women approach sexual encounters are shaped by their sex education, their understanding of male and female desire, and their construction of their self-images (Fine, 1988; Thompson, 1990).

The WRAP data illustrate, as do many other surveys and studies, a particular slant to sex education: too little, too late, too mechanical (Farrell, 1978). While some schools and some teachers are exceptions, the limited and constraining nature of information about sex provided in most British schools lacks almost any content on emotions, sexual relationships or female desire. For these young women, the sexual knowledge offered was almost entirely linked to the mechanics of reproduction. Information was set in the context of science, especially biology, reflecting the medicalization and fragmentation of women's bodies in the broader society. As one young woman commented:

> A: They should do a lot more instead of just pregnancy and contraception, things like that. There's too much pregnancy in the first year, from the third year, pregnancy, pregnancy, pregnancy.

Sex education for young women, both inside and outside school, is frequently couched in a 'protective discourse' (Thomson and Scott, 1991), stressing the dangers that sexual activity can bring in terms of pregnancy and disease, and avoiding the complexity of relationships and the possibilities of pleasure and desire. This education often comes too late for those who are already putting their bodies at risk.

> A: . . . they were just starting to give us sex education, and half the class weren't bloody virgins any more, so they didn't need it.

It can be a problem for teachers and parents that talking about sex threatens to bring the body into young people's consciousness. Sex talk connects the disconnections of gendered disembodiment and gives young people the power to embarrass adults, or be embarrassed by them, by asking about or alluding to their own and the adults' bodily experiences. Confining sex education to technical knowledge of the fragmented body and keeping within a protective discourse avoids this problem.

Knowledge of the body which is required to explore the possibilities of pleasure is often simply omitted from the sex education agenda; the clitoris being absent, for example, from diagrams of the sexual organs. (There is also little evidence that sex education is used to challenge the ways in which young men are taught to think about women's bodies). Masturbation by women, female orgasm or the nature of female sexual pleasure were rarely considered in schools or at home. If masturbation was touched on at all, it was usually in relation to men:

> A: I can't remember, it was something to do with, for men. It was more men they talked about, not women — how they can relieve their sexual feelings without having sex.

One teacher had discussed masturbation in response to a pupil's question:

Q: Was he talking about men masturbating?
A: Mmmm.
Q: Were you ever told at school that women could masturbate?
A: No.

While the route to masculine sexuality might well prove problematic for men (and our accounts from young men suggest that this can be the case), they are provided with an image of male sexual identity in which sex, and their own definition of sexual activity, are legitimized. For men, potentially positive images of male sexuality are widely available, including the legitimation of male desire and a concept of pleasurable sex (albeit defined in a limited way). For young women, in contrast, since female sexuality is strongly associated with reproduction, it is difficult for them to develop a positive image of female sexuality or their own ideas of what might constitute pleasurable sex (Wilton, 1991).

A young woman may be knowledgeable about sexual passion but this knowledge may be defined in terms of servicing men's needs. One young woman illustrates a tension here when she claims a relationship in which each partner gives the other pleasure, but also clearly states that her pleasure is subordinate to his.

Q: What did you expect from sex?
A: Oh, gosh. On — when we do have any kind of sexual activity, for me the — the forefront of my mind is that I want — I want to make him happy, I want to — I — I think, you know, I want to do everything for him, you know, I ask him, 'is there anything I can do for you? 'cos I just really want to make you happy', which is ever so funny 'cos he — he's exactly the same about me, so for me it's making him happy and for him it seems to be making me happy. And I find that if – if I can make – I mean when he actually reaches orgasm, for me that – that can actually override whatever – me - 'cos I think, you know, I've made, you know, that's it, I've – I've made him really happy, and that gives me an amazing feeling, I think that's really great. But no, I certainly don't mind if say I don't have an orgasm, I don't mind that at all.

While we do not denigate the desire and capacity to give happiness, a woman who wants to make her partner happy at the expense of her own desires can be putting her body at risk. Love may lead to communication of desires between partners, but it may equally lead to a romantic sacrifice of her desires. She makes him happy because she loves him, and so she meets what she sees as his needs, and defines her own satisfaction in terms of a general contentment with the relationship, in which her sexual satisfaction is unnecessary. Love as an alternative to shared sexual understanding leads to the pill rather than to protection against infection; to letting him regard her body as his; to his needs defining the encounter. Lover entails trust, and trusting one's partners puts one's own body in their hands. This can make safeguarding the body through safer sexual practices very difficult. Her particular perception of sexual knowledge than feeds the disembodiment which constructs her surface image as separated from her unknowing body and self.

Lacking a materially grounded knowledge of sex and sensuality through recognition of their own bodies, young women adopt the socially prevalent and culturally legitimated substitute of romantic expectations. Having a boyfriend in a socially recognized relationship becomes more valuable than an autonomous female sexuality. To meet these expectations they must also meet the requirements of feminine sexuality, and cultivate a surface inscription of socially acceptable femininity on that same, relatively unknown, and often fiercely criticized body.

Young Women's Self-Images – The Surfaces of Disembodied Femininity

Women are much more likely than men to be dissatisfied with their body and to attempt to change it through dietary regimes and exercise, in efforts to meet the requirements of a fragmented and disembodied femininity (Martin, 1989; Bordo, 1990; McCarthy, 1990).[7] Despite the often consummate skills they develop in constructing this surface representation of femininity (Smith, 1988), these young women are disembodied in the sense of being detached from their sensuality and alienated from their material bodies (Holland *et al.*, 1992b).

There are, at any one time, a limited range of potentially acceptable feminine images, including those specific to different cultural and sub-cultural groups, upon which young women can draw and which they can help to create.[8] The images which they devise within these social constraints, however, may be understood differently by the young women from the way in which they are read by the men who view them. *A skilful representation of self as sexually knowing might be produced* by a young woman, who is in fact unknowing.

This disjunction between knowledge and self-image may lead a young woman into sexually unsafe situations. Situations are unsafe where something is expected of her, a sexual or sexualized encounter, which she does not understand, or for which she is not prepared. Young women spend a good deal of time on their outward appearance in order to construct a female body which will act as a magnet to attract men, but they may have little control over who they attract, and the sexual expectations that they are then supposed to meet. One young woman in the sample, who was not sexually active, identified herself as shy in relation to men, and was opposed to sex before marriage on religious grounds. On at least two occasions, men with whom she was having a conversation had suggested to her that she was 'not a virgin'. She could not understand why they had this perception of her.

Young women must manage their appearance very carefully in order to stay on the right side of the slippery boundary between being acceptably attractive and overly sexualized. They learn that in order to be acceptable to men they must control their bodies; they must be vigilant against fat, spots and surplus hair; against evidence of menstruation; against anything which might break up the smooth surface of the feminine body.

> Q: Had you not really thought about going out with boys before then?
> A: Yes, but I was quite fat and I lost weight when I was about fifteen, sixteen.
> Q: Did you feel that [being fat] excluded you?
> A: Yes.

There is a lack of congruence between the control which is exercised by young women over the surfaces and contours of the body, and the limited knowledge and lack of control over what happens both within the body and at the interface between male and female bodies.

There is a related disengagement between the surface image of the body (the way femininity is socially inscribed on the body) and the young women's sense of self. This was demonstrated in responses to a direct question in the interview asking the young women what their image of themselves was. In no instance did they respond in terms of a physical image. In general they had difficulty in answering this question at all but, when they did manage to do so, tended to speak of their 'personality' or 'character' or what their friends thought of these. These responses were given in cases where, to the interviewer, a tremendous amount of careful thought and energy appeared to have been invested in their physical presentation of self. Some of these young women were training to be beauty therapists, and our field notes refer to the extreme version of manicured and depilated femininity which they presented.

Young women can become conscious of their image as a construction when they make a distinction between the presentation of themselves that men are respond to, and what they think of as their 'real self'.

> A: Oh, yeah. I mean at first like some of the people used to say, 'oh you're so nice and so gorgeous, you look so nice all the time', and at first I thought, 'oh, my God, it's so amazing', and then after a while it meant nothing. Like, 'yeah, you see this, but what am I really like, you know, who cares, you don't care'.

> A: I think with other boyfriends, I think Anne (her friend) found this as well, is that they like you when you're sweet and you're beautiful and, you know, whatever, you've got a new outfit on or whatever, whatever reason, but as soon as you feel depressed or down in the dumps or — I don't know, got a sudden rush of acne or something, they just don't want to know.

The power of masculine privilege in sexual encounters is often recognized by young women, at least in terms of the 'double standard', but the extent to which they contribute to the reproduction of this power through their own femininity is much less clear to them. The surface image of the feminine body is literally made-up every day, constructed to be socially acceptable, sexually desirable, or otherwise, in the here and now. This location in the immediate present, combined with restricted knowledge of the possibilities of sexuality and the disembodiment which characterizes the representation of femininity, leaves many young women unprepared to become sexual, or to recognize themselves as sexual. One consequence can be a 'reality gap' between expectations and experience recognized by so many in the behaviour of young women. Their gendered understanding of sexuality can lead them to treat pregnancy and disease as events which cannot possibly happen to them.[9] Two young women had not thought of using contraception, because they had not considered that they could be at risk of pregnancy or disease.

> Q: Were you using condoms then or –
> A: No.
> Q: You weren't? Never?

A: No. Didn't think of it.

Q: Yeah.

A: Well the first time we didn't think of it, after — because it struck me after I got pregnant . . .

A: I kept saying it wouldn't happen to me, it could happen to anybody else but not me, and it's like — such a shock [she went for a pregnancy test and rang the doctor for the result] and he just said it was positive. It was like — I don't know, it was just like everything just stood still. It was like — I just couldn't believe it.

The shock caused this young woman to insist on condom use in her next sexual encounter, but she found this a strange and difficult task:[10]

A: It's made me a lot wiser now, a lot more careful, I slept with somebody and like, first I said, 'condom — get it out', sort of thing. It's like — it's the first — I don't know, it's never really occurred to me, I don't know why, it just suddenly fell out, like, 'use that — otherwise'. It just felt really strange to come out and say it, and I thought, well you've got to say it, for your own peace of mind.

Both these young women decided to have abortions with no reference to the wishes of the potential fathers. But in their sexual relationships they were still largely dependent on the way the men they were with defined the sexual encounter. The moulding of their surface images and the disciplining of their bodies distances them from their own sexuality, and so from caring for their bodily safety.

The Exercise of Control and the Elusive Body

Braidotti (1991) suggests that the process of getting to know and of getting to control the embodied self are one and the same, and it is our contention that the particular kind of knowledge about their bodies that feminine young women most easily have access to can result in them having less control than men in their sexual encounters. They appear to be in control of their bodies, and may feel in control, but they can also lose control, and so lose touch with their desires. Struggling to live up to idealized images of femininity can lead to the disciplining of docile bodies.

Our data suggest that where women have lacked control in relation to their bodies they may develop strategies to gain more control. Extreme cases illustrate the contradictions of control/loss of control in women's attempts to govern their bodies. Starving is a drastic measure which women can use to deny the sexuality of the body. Anorexia nervosa is an exercise in the apparent control of a material body which is in fact out of control. This can be seen as taking the control of femininity to extremes, expressing resistance and restraint in the same gesture (Bordo, 1989).

Abstaining from sexual relations by choosing celibacy is another possible strategy for controlling the body. One of our respondents, who had lost control of her body through the violence of being raped, had not only given up sex with men, but had also altered her whole surface appearance in order to discourage their advances.

> A: It [the rape] was a very important thing in my life, it's changed me. I used to be a real right one of the girls. I used to wear high heels all the time, and now it really changed me. It changed me in a lot of positive ways I think. Yes, women should be able to wear what they want but they're not. I'm not going to wear the uniform of a bimbo and be treated like one.

This particular young woman seemed comfortable with her decision, and at the time seemed to be more interested in establishing her autonomy than in sexual relationships with men.

Another of our respondents, who had been sexually abused by her father, disliked sex and tended to avoid it, but was unhappy with her lack of control in this situation. She faced the problem of how to care for her body while distanced from it through her distaste for sex. She had been in a relationship with a boy from the age of thirteen until she was seventeen but there had been no sex until she was sixteen and a half when her boyfriend began to want a sexual relationship. She gave in to him because she was afraid of losing him but she hated the sexual intercourse.

> A: I felt awful. I remember crying and saying I just can't do it. It was the worst thing, it was awful.

The relationship, which was what she had wanted, continued for six months at the cost of her having sex, which she did not want.

> Q: So you split up after he went to university?

A: Yes, and I felt awful about having slept with him.

Q: What, after you split up?

A: I just felt dirty in a way.

Q: Because it hadn't really developed into anything more?

A: No. I feel that — a bit different, but I felt that after I split up with my boyfriend I felt a bit dirty having had sex and everything and then leaving me.

She was currently trying to regain control of her sexuality in a new sexual relationship, but although she described it as good in other ways, she still felt that she got nothing out of sex.

A: It just seems to me that you are there for men and I just can't believe it. I think that a lot of girls feel as though they are there just for the men's satisfaction, they don't feel as though they are being fulfilled in any way. They are just there to excite men.

Since women are capable of resisting masculine power, even relatively inexperienced young women could develop some control through gaining positive knowledge of the body and understanding of their own pleasure. This was not, though, a common experience in this age group (Holland *et al.*, 1992a). Positive experiences seemed to come from being able to talk about and feel comfortable with the material body, menstruation, sensuality, desires, in the context of a sexual relationship. Given these conditions, a young woman could be taken unawares by orgasm.

A: And then, you know, I came — when I came up last August, going out with David, the sex has just been the most wonderful, fantastic experience I've ever had with him.

Q: So that must have been a real -

A: It was, I mean blimey -

Q: — surprise.

A: — I didn't realize it could be like this, it was just it's — I've just never ever been unhappy or unsatisfied with anything we've done together.

Q: So what's made it different with David?

A: I think — I've lost — I've grown a lot of self-confidence, I mean before I wouldn't let anybody — I had to be under the sheets all the time, I wouldn't let anybody see me and I — I certainly wouldn't walk around the room naked, which is what I do sometimes, you know, together, I don't worry about that now. It — it's just the way that he was with me. I mean he was a lot more experienced than me to start with, so there wasn't any sort of silly fumbling around and he — there was a lot more communication than there was — we talked to each other before, how we were playing about, messing around, we'd actually talk about it beforehand.

Another young woman made an explicit link between sexual pleasure, feeling confident and being able to communicate with a partner.

Q: So you were all aware that women could have orgasms?
A: Oh yeah, we knew, but we didn't know what it was.
Q: So how did you move on from that? Was it going out with an older person or what?
A: I think it was because of Lee really. Just like spending so much time with somebody you could talk about what you like best, and what you didn't like. 'And if you do this that makes it better for me' and 'if I do this to you, do you like that?' sort of thing. So –
Q: Actually being able to talk about sex –
A: Being able to be confident of someone, to actually talk about it and not get all embarrassed. If I'm embarrassed I can't say anything. And it's only since then really.
Q: That gives you the sense that you're in a more equal position.
A: And you're older anyway so don't think it's as embarrassing. It was awful. I used to think about it.

This management of intimacy could increase with sexual experience and with age, but not necessarily. Neither age nor experience will ensure sexual pleasure or safety if a young woman defines the feminine body as subordinate to men's needs.

A: . . . I've only slept with, is it five, six people. I still don't know whether I'm doing it right, do you know what I mean? Lie back and think of England. I mean I do sometimes. I think it helps — I don't know what to do or anything — I'd like experience, yeah, I'd definitely like experience. I'd like someone actually to tell me whether I'm doing it right or wrong.

If she expects men to define what is appropriate, pleasurable and permissible in sexual encounters, she will control her body by disciplining it into femininity, but in becoming alienated from it will relinquish control of her own sexual safety.

Challenging Sexual Risk

Women have long been expected to contain and control male sexuality (Bland, 1982) and this has been reinforced in the context of HIV and AIDS (Waldby *et al.*, 1990). Much health education material aimed at heterosexuals, in the UK and elsewhere, has focused on the need for women to take control in sexual encounters.[11] This expectation both ignores the dynamics of gendered power embedded in sexual relations and assumes a degree of engagement with bodily practices which is beyond the experience of many young women. Much of our data stands in contradiction to the impression given in some magazines of a new generation of sexually assertive young women in tune with their bodies and ready to ask men to give them what they want.[12] Women's control over their own bodies, their concern for sexual safety, and their agency in asserting a positive female sexuality are situated in cultural contexts in which female bodies need to be corrected, controlled and remodelled to constitute desirable images of femininity.

The social inequalities between men and women in sexual encounters do not rule out the possibility of women's resistance, agency, desire, pleasure, empowerment. We do not wish to imply that men always oppress women, and our initial analysis of data from young men shows that they can find negotiating sexual encounters difficult and uncertain, particularly in making the first moves. They can be surprised by women. But the social construction of femininity and masculinity, however fragile, contested and unstable these constructions might be, systematically privileges masculinity over femininity, and in silencing female sexual desire, privileges men's sexual 'needs' over women's sexual safety. Sex can be an unnecessarily negative experience for young women because of the appropriation of female desire in the construction of heterosexual sexuality.

While Foucault's conception of the body can be used to challenge claims for the fixity of women's sexuality and to deconstruct patriarchal power, our data suggest that this view cannot take adequate account of women's experience of the specificity and complexity of their sexuality. Heterosexual femininity is both material and a contradictory construction which draws women into working for their own subordination. The disembodied femininity which results help to reproduce male sexual power and to put women's bodies at risk. Women's successful construction and disciplining of their bodies as feminine reproduces their bodies as sexually desirable material for subordinating to men's sexual needs, whether or not women or men are aware of this, or want this. The fragmentation and medicalization of women's bodies, which is characteristic of sex education discourse, is poor preparation for effective control of sexual safety. We do not mean that all women lose control of their bodies so that they are always at risk, nor that women are the only losers. Achieving pleasurable sex, however, does not in itself confront institutionalized male power or the risks of male violence.

Women can of course grasp their own embodiment and take control of their own sexuality by recognizing femininity as limited, restrictive and unsafe. Knowledge and experience of sexual pleasure can connect a woman with her body in ways which challenge disembodied femininity and so make her assertion of a need for safer sex more practicable. But where women's self-esteem, self-image, self-knowledge and emotional needs are tied to a highly skilled but limited social construction of femininity, then women will continue to support men's power and their own subordination. The assertion of a need to take care of their bodies through safer sexual practices by young women challenges the disembodied femininity of conventional heterosexuality, and exposes the body as still a contested site.

Notes

1 Anthropology has always paid heed to the cultural meanings inscribed on the body, but only recently to the gendered meanings of such inscription.
2 While we are using the term 'women' generally here we do not intend to imply that social divisions (e.g. race/ethnicity, class, sexual orientation, ablebodiedness) between women are not socially, politically and personally significant, but that elements of socially constructed sexuality are shared. We have found no significant differences in gendered experience of sexual encounters across the boundaries of class, race/ethnicity or physical challenge. We would argue that the social construction of heterosexuality differs empirically from the social construction of lesbianism. The question of the nature and extent of cultural variations in sexuality are not yet well established (Caplan, 1987).
3 The Women, Risk and AIDS Project is staffed by the authors and Sue Sharpe working collectively, and has been financed by a two-year grant from the ESRC. It has also received grants from Goldsmiths' College Research Fund and the Department of Health. Valuable assistance has been given by Jane Preston, Polly Radcliffe and Janet Ransom. WRAP used a purposive sample to interview in depth 150 young women aged 16-21 in London and Manchester between 1988 and 1990, and has additional data from 500 questionnaires. The Leverhulme Trust gave a further one-year grant for a study of young men in 1991-2, and for comparison of the two studies. Tim Rhodes was a team member on this project.

4   There is considerable support for this view. For example, Mathieu (1979) argues radically for the social nature of maternity; Edholm (1982) gives examples of the social definition of the biological, and a range of issues are raised by contributors to Caplan (1987).

5   Foucault thinks of people in terms of subjects or bodies who have no essential or fixed truth as to what they 'really' are, but who are constituted by the particular discourses (e.g. clinical medicine, history, education theory) of their time which define what is allowed to be true. By discourse (or discursive practices) he means not simply ways of talking, but the interrelated rules of what is taken to be true, permitted, taken for granted in the human sciences (Foucault, 1991).

6   A problem with Foucault's position is that it can lead to plural feminisms and political relativism in which feminism has not particular political object (Fraser, 1989; Nicholson, 1990). Women of different ethnicities, classes, abilities and sexual orientations are left to work out their own forms of liberation. They can do their own thing in resisting discourses without having to pay political attention to the paradox of being both deeply socially divided from other women, but also united by socially constructed sexuality in relation to men's gendered power.

7   In the UK, Hill (1992, p. 430) notes: 'Dissatisfaction with body size and shape is growing in both the number of people who experience it, and the distance they are from the ideal'. This dissatisfaction has spread to children, giving a high level of dissatisfaction with body weight among 9-to-12-year-olds and the early emergence of unrealistic body weight preferences linked to low self-esteem in girls (Hill *et al.*, 1992).

8   An interesting version of this creation of sub-cultural femininity came with the subversion by female punks of the more conventional artefacts of femininity. Their torn clothing, with make-up and hairstyle designed to shock, signified an alienated and resistant group identity. It could also be seen as contradictory. These subversive feminine images could take as long to construct as the more traditional versions and, when spread more widely than in their initial, politicized form, be as distant and disembodied from the selves 'inside' too. Some questions could also be asked about the change in the presentation of the female in the current rave scene. Here women's style appears to be moving from the loose, baggy unisex clothing for men and women to form-fitting lycra for women (*The Guardian*, 2 April 1992).

9   See Abrams *et al.* (1990) for a discussion of young people's feelings of invulnerability in relation to AIDS.

10 The contradictions and unpredictability of condom use are explored in Holland *et al.* (1991).

11 An 'America Responds to AIDS' campaign poster states, 'if he doesn't have a condom, you just have to take a deep breath and tell him to go get one'. The UK campaign directed at young heterosexuals states, 'she is too embarrassed to ask him to use a condom. What's your excuse?'

12 *Company*, March and April 1992. The *Elle*/Durex sex survey (Alexander, 1992) also presents a picture of a proud new woman who treats sex as a playground rather than a battleground, making the first approaches to men and demanding satisfying sex on her own terms. But Alexander adds: 'Inevitably the picture is not uniformly positive' and, despite the growing number of women talking control of their bodies, she also reports 'grim tales' of regret, anger and ignorance.

References

ABRAMS, D., ABRAHAM, C., SPEARS, R. and MARKS, D. (1990) 'AIDS invulnerability; relationships, sexual behaviour and attitudes among 16–19 year-olds, in AGGLETON,

P., DAVIES, P. and HART, G. (Eds) *AIDS: Individual, Cultural and Policy Dimensions*, London: The Falmer Press.

ALEXANDER, J. (1992) 'Sex: The Results of our Survey', Elle, April.

BARRETT, M. (1991) *The Politics of Truth: From Marx to Foucault*, Cambridge, Polity Press.

BARTKY, S.L. (1990) *Femininity and Domination: Studies in the Phenomenology of Oppression*, London, Routledge.

BLAND, L. (1982) '"Guardians of the Race" or "Vampires upon the Nation's Health"?: Female Sexuality and its Regulation in Early Twentieth-Century Britain', in WHITELEGG, E. *et al.* (Eds) *The Changing Experience of Women*, Oxford, Martin Robertson/Open University.

BORDO, S. (1989) 'The Body and the Reproduction of Femininity: A Feminist Appropriation of Foucault', in JAGGAR, A. AND BORDO, S. (Eds) *Gender/Body/Knowledge: Feminist Reconstructions of Being and Knowing*, New Brunswick: Rutgers University Press.

BORDO, S. (1990) 'Material Girl: The Effacements of Postmodern Culture', *Michigan Quarterly Review*, Fall, pp. 653–76.

BRAIDOTTI, R. (1991) *Patterns of Dissonance*, Cambridge, Polity Press.

CAPLAN, P. (Ed.) (1987) *The Cultural Construction of Sexuality*, London, Tavistock.

DWORKIN, A. (1988) 'Dangerous and Deadly', *Trouble and Strife*, 14, pp. 42–5.

EDHOLM, F. (1982) 'The Unnatural Family', in WHITELEGG, E. *et al.* (Eds) *The Changing Experience of Women*, Oxford, Martin Robertson/Open University.

FARRELL, C. with KELLAHER, L. (1978) *My Mother Said . . . The Way Young People Learned About Sex and Birth Control*, London, Routledge and Kegan Paul.

FEATHERSTONE, M., HEPWORTH, M. and TURNER, B.S. (Eds) (1991) *The Body: Social Process and Cultural Theory*, London, Sage.

FINE, M. (1988) 'Sexuality, Schooling, and Adolescent Females: The Missing Discourse of Desire', *Harvard Educational Review*, 58, 1, pp. 29–53.

FOUCAULT, M. (1980a) 'The History of Sexuality' in FOUCAULT, M. *Power/Knowledge* (Ed. C. Gordon), London, Harvester.

FOUCAULT, M. (1980b) 'The Confession of the Flesh', in FOUCAULT, M. *Power/Knowledge*, (Ed. C. Gordon), London, Harvester.

FOUCAULT, M. (1988) *Politics, Philosophy, Culture: Interviews and Other Writings* (Ed. L.D. Kritzman), London, Routledge.

FOUCAULT, M. (1991) 'Politics and the Study of Discourse', in BURCHELL, G., GORDON, C. and MILLER, P. (Eds) *The Foucault Effect: Studies in Governmentality*, London, Harvester Wheatsheaf.

FRASER, N. (1989) *Unruly Practices: Power, Discourse and Gender in Contemporary Social Theory*, Cambridge, Polity Press.

GATENS, M. (1988) 'Towards a Feminist Philosophy of the Body', in CAINE, B., GROSZ, E.A. and LEPERVANCHE, M. DE, (Eds) *Crossing Boundaries: Feminisms and the Critique of Knowledge*, Sydney, Allen and Unwin.

GROSZ, E. (1990) 'Inscriptions and Body-Maps: Representation and the Corporeal', in THREADGOLD, T. and CRANNY-FRANCIS, A. (Eds) *Feminine, Masculine and Representation*, London, Allen and Unwin.

HARTSOCK, N. (1983) *Money, Sex and Power: Toward a Feminist Historical Materialism*, London, Longman.

HEKMAN, S. (1990) *Gender and Knowledge: Elements of a Postmodern Feminism*, Boston, Northeastern University Press.

HILL, A.J. (1992) 'Fear and Loathing of Obesity: The Rise of Dieting in Childhood', in AILHAUD, G., GUY-GRAND, B., LAFONTON, M. and RICQUIER, D. (Eds) *Obesity in Europe 91*, London, John Libbey.

HILL, A.J., JONES, E. and STACK, J. (1992) 'A Weight on Children's Minds: Body Shape Dissatisfactions at 9-Years Old', Paper presented to *Annual Conference of the British Psychological Society*, Scarborough.

HITE, S. (1987) *Women and Love*, London, Penguin.

HOLLAND, J., RAMAZANOGLU, C., SCOTT, S., SHARPE, S. and THOMSON, R. (1991) 'Between Embarrassment and Trust: Young Women and the Diversity of Condom Use' in AGGLETON, P., HART, G. and DAVIES, P. (Eds) *AIDS: Responses, Interventions and Care*, London, Falmer Press.

HOLLAND, J., RAMAZANOGLU, C., SCOTT, S., SHARPE, S. and THOMSON, R. (1992a) 'Pressure, Resistance, Empowerment: Young Women and the Negotiation of Safer Sex', in AGGLETON, P., HART, G. and DAVIES, P. (Eds) *AIDS: Rights, Risk and Reason*, London, Falmer Press.

HOLLAND, J., RAMAZANOGLU, C., SHARPE, S. and THOMSON, R. (1992b) 'Power and Desire: The Embodiment of Female Sexuality', paper to be presented at the First International Conference on Girls and Girlhood, Amsterdam, June 1992.

HOLLAND, J., RAMAZANOGLU, C., SHARPE, S. and THOMSON, R. (1992c) 'Men's Needs and Women's Agency: Social Constraints on Young Women's Sexual Safety', *Sociological Review*, in press.

LATHER, P. (1991) *Getting Smart: Feminist Research and Pedagogy with/in the Postmodern*, London, Routledge.

MCCARTHY, M. (1990) 'The Thin Ideal, Depression and Eating Disorders in Women', *Behaviour, Research and Therapy*, vol. 28, no. 3, pp. 205-15.

MARTIN, E. (1989) *The Woman in the Body*, Milton Keynes, Open University Press.

MATHIEU, N-C. (1979) 'Biological Paternity, Social Maternity: On Abortion and Infanticide as Unrecognised Indicators of the Cultural Character for Maternity' in HARRIS, C.C. (Ed.) *The Sociology of the Family*, Sociological Review Monograph 28.

MORRIS, M. (1979) 'The Pirate's Fiancée', in MORRIS, M. and PATTON, P. (Eds) *Michel Foucault: Power, Truth, Strategy*, Sydney, Feral Publications.

NICHOLSON, L. (Ed.) (1990) *Feminism/Postmodernism*, London, Routledge.

SAWICKI, J. (1991) *Disciplining Foucault: Feminism, Power and the Body*, London, Routledge.

SCHOR, N. (1987) 'Dreaming Dissymmetry: Barthes, Foucault and Sexual Difference' in JARDINE, A. and SMITH, P. (Eds) *Men in Feminism*, London, Methuen.

SCOTT, S. and MORGAN, D. (1992) 'Bodies in a Social Landscape' in MORGAN, D. and SCOTT, S. (Eds) *Body Matters: Essays on the Sociology of the Body*, London, Falmer Press.

SMITH, D. (1988) 'Femininity as Discourse', in ROMAN, L.G. and CHRISTIAN-SMITH, L.K. with ELLSWORTH, E. (Eds) *Becoming Feminine*, London, Falmer Press.

THOMSON, R. and SCOTT, S. (1991) *Learning About Sex: Young Women and the Social Construction of Sexual Identity* (WRAP Paper 4), London, Tufnell Press.

THOMPSON, S. (1990) 'Putting a Big Thing into a Little Hole: Teenage Girls' Accounts of Sexual Initiation', *The Journal of Sex Research*, vol. 27, no. 3, pp. 341-61.

TURNER, B. (1984) *The Body and Society*, Oxford, Blackwell.

WALDBY, C., KIPPAX, S. and CRAWFORD, J. (1990) 'Theory in the Bedroom: A Report from the Macquarie University AIDS and Heterosexuality Project', *Australian Journal of Social Issues*, vol. 25, no. 3, pp. 177-85.

WILTON, T. (1991) 'Feminism and the Erotics of Health Promotion', paper given at the Fifth Conference on the Social Aspects of AIDS, London.

Chapter 5

Feminism and the Erotics of Health Promotion

Tamsin Wilton

> There are *no* valid generalisations to be made about sex and women's lives except for the central fact that we are all hungry for the power of desire and we are all terribly, deeply afraid.
> (Dorothy Allison, 1984)

The association of eroticism with health promotion is a phenomenon which has become very much taken for granted in the context of HIV and AIDS.[1] It is easy to forget that it is still very much a novel practice, as yet inadequately theorized. The idea of the Health Education Authority explicitly promoting masturbation as good for your health would have been unimaginable a mere decade ago, as would the prospect of Princess Diana shaking hands with 'known homosexuals'. There is much to applaud in the apparent challenge to sexual hypocrisy necessitated by AIDS. Yet we should be wary of rejoicing too soon. AIDS, as Jeffrey Weeks warns us, has become 'a battleground for defining the sort of culture we are and want to become' (Weeks, 1990). As both Foucauldian and feminist analyses suggest, the body, in particular the sexualized body, is a key site for the disputation and contestation of meaning and of political power. Preventing the sexual transmission of HIV intimately involves the exercise of power, specifically power over one's own body, and power to negotiate as an equal during any sexual encounter. Neither power nor sex are 'natural', rather, they are socially and discursively constituted and assigned, in a process which is profoundly gendered and inequitable. My suggestion is that we ignore the constitutive power of discourses of sex and sexuality at our peril. As Janet Holland and her colleagues insist, 'Health education policy will not be effective if the imbalance of power in the social construction of sexuality is not understood and acted upon' (Holland *et al.*, 1990b, p. 23).

The task of promoting safer sex, still our only strategy in preventing the sexual transmission of HIV, demands that we develop appropriate practices of representation of the sexual. Representation has always been a key site of sexual politics, of the struggle for control of sexual meaning and definition. Sexualized body imagery has long been exploited in the marketplace, and feminist critiques have demonstrated the constitutive power of such sexualized representation in the oppression of women (Davies *et al.*, 1987; Pollock, 1987; Williamson, 1987). Safer sex promotional materials too are increasingly exploiting sexualized body imagery, though the product is sex itself, or more specifically a particular group of sexual practices which constitute safer sex. The other key representational practice which sells sex in this way is pornography. It is inevitable that, by adopting representational practices which seek to eroticize safer sex, discourses of HIV/AIDS health promotion are inevitably allied with discourses of pornography, a 'marriage' by no means unproblematic in the context of the sexual politics of representation. It is crucial to the promotion of safer sex that we recognize that safer sex materials themselves intersect with and impact upon pre-existing discourses of sexuality which, in addition to having a perceived political–representational role in both sexual and gender politics also have a constitutive role in the construction of sexuality and desire itself.

In this chapter I shall question the putatively radical assertion that safer sex materials must be erotic in order to be successful (Patton, 1985), and that what Simon Watney (1987) calls 'a pornographic healing' represents the only oppositional discourse available to us to challenge the oppressive social and cultural practices of heterosexism and the power of the homophobic state. I shall interrogate safer sex promotional strategies from a feminist poststructuralist position, and show that, far from being in opposition to the successful promotion of safer sex, a feminist critique of pornography and of safer sex discourse itself is essential both to the medical struggle against HIV, and the social and political struggle against AIDS.

Feminism Identified as Antagonistic to Safer Sex Promotion

At a national conference held in 1990 in Manchester on the theme of 'AIDS, HIV and Civil Liberties', pornography was alluded to in a workshop on health education. That workshop recommended that 'the debate on pornography or obscenity legislation must be pursued energetically, with the central focus being to preserve freedom for the promotion of safer sex information, rather than on particular feminist ideologies' (Manchester City Council, 1990). This apparent antagonism of feminist ideology to the promotion of safer sex information depends on a depressingly familiar wilful misrepresentation of the feminist critique of pornography. Those who defend pornography, and they include feminists among others, suggest that a critique of pornography is an attack on civil liberties (Rodgerson and Semple, 1990; Ellis *et al.*, 1990; Kaveney, 1990) or an expression of femine erotophobia (Jeffreys, 1987; Cole, 1989; Watney, 1987). They misrepresent the feminist critique of pornography as a rejection of all 'sexually explicit material' (Jeffreys, 1987; MacKinnon, 1989; Rodgerson and Semple, 1990). Ironically, by chosing to define pornography simplistically as sexually explicit material, sexual libertarianism merely reflects, and hence reinforces, right-wing moralism. Both discourses, by this semantic collusion, limit any political critique of pornography to purely moral notions of corruption and perversion which posit sexual subjectivity as essential and 'given'.

The radical feminist critique of pornography is quite different, focusing on the representation of the sexual subordination of women to men (Jeffreys, 1987; Brownmiller, 1975; Dworkin, 1988; Cole, 1989; Allison, 1984). It is neither sexually explicit material, nor sexually arousing material, which is identified as oppressive to women (Brownmiller, 1975; MacKinnon, 1989; Dworkin, 1988; Jeffreys, 1990; Cole, 1989). Rather, it is the recognition of pornography's discursive structuration of both female and male desire and subjectivity, and the part that process plays in the establishment and maintenance of the gendered power relations inherent in heteropatriarchal culture (Gavey, 1990; Weedon, 1987; MacKinnon, 1989).

The Sex-Positive 'Alternative'

Any health promotion strategy must engage with issues of identity, with culture, and with community if it is to be effective, even in persuading people to change their diet (Homans and Aggleton, 1988; Patton 1990b). HIV/AIDS health promotion is faced with the added difficulty of having to address that most intimate and defended area of subjectivity, sexuality. Issues of sexual identity, the body, its desires and acts are foregrounded by HIV/AIDS, and must be confronted within discourses of health promotion and social policy as never before (Frutchey, 1990; Patton, 1990b; Watney, 1990a). Additionally, HIV and AIDS have demanded recognition of the diversity of sexual constituencies within what had previously been assumed to be relatively discrete social groups.

We may no longer safely assume that men are either gay or straight, nor that men who have sex with men necessarily identify as gay or bisexual. HIV/AIDS health promotion has therefore evolved into a complexity of targeting, with specific material aimed at increasingly specialized sexual groups. Such targeting practices are themselves, of course, active in the discursive constitution of subjectivity and of sex itself, something which will be further explored below.

Many have argued that the most appropriate strategy to ensure widespread adoption of safer sexual practices, whether this means condom use or alternatives to penetration, is to 'eroticize safer sex' (Watney, 1987; Patton, 1990a, 1990b). Watney, indeed, explicitly identifies pornography as *the only* means of establishing the practice of safer sex, by working 'at the level of fantasy'. Whilst it is doubtless true that fantasy is a core component of sexual subjectivity, we need to recognize that 'fantasy expresses ideology, it is not exempt from it' (MacKinnon, 1989). Acknowledging that fantasy is, therefore, available for deconstruction, and that the erotic is only recently the province of health promotion, it is necessary to interrogate notions of sexual identity, sexual pleasure, risk and sexual desire as they are constituted both in dominant heteropatriarchal discourse and within the discursive practices of HIV/AIDS health promotion.

Sexual Identity

Faced with AIDS, heteropatriarchal discourse is compelled to defend masculinity, that unquestionable hegemonic norm to which all else is 'other', against contamination, both literal and metaphorical. So, as Roberta McGrath has described, 'both heterosexual women and gay men are pathologised as reservoirs of disease — as degenerate and dangerous' (McGrath, 1990). The early stages of the epidemic in Britain witnessed the unpleasant phenomenon of widespread media homophobia, which, by labelling AIDS as the just deserts of the perverted and the promiscuous, lulled the (presumptively heterosexual and monogamous) general public into a deadly sense of security. Lynne Segal writes, 'The onset of AIDS gave (the) pro-family, anti-sexual permissiveness rhetoric an apparent legitimacy, not simply in the name of conservative morality but also in the name of medical wisdom' (Segal, 1990). The prevailing, all too familiar, text might be summed up as 'the wages of sin is death', the sin in question being all forms of sex perceived as outside the heterosexual, monogamous familial 'norm'. Watney has characterized this as a 'crisis of representation', which he sees as putting the gay identity itself at risk

(Watney, 1987, 1990b), whilst Paula Treichler has demanded an 'epidemiology of signification' as the first step in a radical response to AIDS (Treichler, 1987).

Sex has never been politically neutral. The traditional binary divide of the personal and the political, long recognized by feminism as illusory, vanishes utterly when scrutinizing the relationship between sex and the state. As Foucault recognized, 'sex has become a focal point of the exercise of power through the discursive constitution of the body' (Foucault, 1978). One key site of struggle for control of sexual meaning is representation. By controlling how sex is represented, the state attempts to control sexuality, policing the bounds of the visible in order to police desire itself. The attack on representations of gay sex may be read as part of the attempt to eradicate homosexual desire altogether from the body politic. As Watney succinctly puts it, 'Censorship sets a cordon sanitaire around lesbians and gay men in Britain' (Watney, 1987). The definition of gay sex as obscene and unlawful has undoubtedly resulted in the unnecessary HIV-related deaths of heterosexuals as well as gay men. The then Chief Medical Officer of the Department of Health was obliged to have copies of American gay magazines, the only source of safer sex information available to him, smuggled in via the diplomatic bag, and obscenity legislation has frequently impeded free and open access to safer sex information (Watney, 1987).

Confronted with the deeply homophobic ideological rhetoric of the state, appalled by its cynical and inhumane 'catpure' of AIDS, it is clearly essential to develop an anti-oppressive, affirmative and empowering alternative. It is perhaps unsurprising that, in reaction to the erotophobia which gleefully proclaims that sex is death, an oppositional discourse has developed which posits not only a sexual identity constructed around sexual activity, and in some cases, specific sexual practices (Patton, 1990a; Dowsett, 1991), but a simplistic elision of sex and life itself. Yet my argument is that this apparently radical, apparently 'sex-positive', liberatory discourse is in fact deeply reactionary, colluding with rather than challenging the hegemony of dominant discourses of the sexual which are oppressive to women and to gay men, and profoundly inimical to the widespread adoption of safer sex. It is also my contention that current practices of representation in HIV/AIDS health promotion which take sexual identity as their focus are themselves counter-productive, acting to perpetuate the hegemony of heterosexual patriarchy and hence to impede the practice of safer sex.

There is, firstly, the problematic issue of 'heterosexual identity' which, as I have argued elsewhere, is an identity largely constructed by negative reference to the 'other'. To be heterosexual is to be 'not like that', that is, not homosexual (Wilton and Aggleton, 1991). Additionally, the hegemony of heterosexuality is predicated upon its status as presumptive norm. Its discursive power lies in the very fact that it is assumed with a totality which pre-empts both challenge and, paradoxically, the need for self-definition. Heterosexuality is not primarily experienced as a sexual identity but rather as something inherent in being human. It is perfectly possible to assume oneself to be heterosexual and yet never engage with issues of sexual desire (Rule, 1985). There are exceptions to this. 'Adolescence', for example, is a social category discursively constructed around notions of the development of a (hetero-)sexual self (Wilton and Aggleton, 1990). Thus 'young people' are recognized as an appropriate heterosexual 'target audience' for the promotion of safer sex.

A second and fundamental problem is that HIV/AIDS health promotion has failed to identify and engage with the interaction between the social construction of gender and the social construction of sexuality. Dominant discourses of gender differentially constitute feminine and masculine sexual subjectivity. To men are allocated sexual desire, the power to choose or reject sexual partners, the power to insist on sexual gratification, ownership of sexual 'drive'. To women are allocated the responsibility for sexual attractiveness, the responsibility for male sexual gratification, the responsibility for sexual responsiveness and the responsibility to *defend themselves against sex* on many levels. Reference to a couple of safer sex leaflets will illustrate how this discourse permeates and is reinforced by HIV/AIDS representational practice. One, the infamous 'sex' leaflet produced by the Terrence Higgins Trust, bears a suggestive drawing of a nude, white, hunky man on the front cover, his modesty protected by the word 'sex'. This represents what is by now a cliché of health promotion, the use of nude or scantily clad hunks to sell safe sex to gay men. The other, produced by a local health authority, is aimed at women, and has a cover devoid of graphic titillation, depending entirely on variety in typeface to attract the punters. Conspicuous on this cover is the warning 'The advice in this leaflet is explicit. Please do not read it if you are easily offended'. (Both leaflets are reproduced in Wilton, 1992.)

What is at work here is a complexity of discursive practices which act to reinforce one another. Gay men, already discursively constructed as sexually active by reason of their gender, are additionally constructed as essentially *sexual* by reason of their membership of a social group defined by its sexuality. This particular text offers no challenge to either discourse, despite the fact that both are oppressive. Indeed, on the front cover of this particular leaflet, gay man has become a sign signifying sex! Women, in contrast, are constructed as having nothing whatever to do with sex, indeed, as finding any mention of sex offensive. This is in direct collusion with pornography, in its feminist sense, as 'a practice of sexual politics, an institution of gender inequality' (MacKinnon, 1989). Pornography is a practice of representation which dispossesses women of the power of sexual definition (MacKinnon, 1989), indeed, of desire itself. By differentially assigning desire to women and to men, by misrepresenting female sexual pleasure as inherently masochistic, pornography is a 'core constitutive process of gender inequality' (MacKinnon, 1989). In other words, the key problem in pornography is not sex, but gender.

An additional problem for health promotional strategies which aim to use sexual identity as a 'hook to grab people's attention' (Frutchey, 1990) is the contested relationship between identity and practice. The social ascription of masculinity demands that biological males achieve masculinity through a variety of actions, central to which is penetrating women sexually (Jeffreys, 1990). Similarly, the imperative of heterosexuality to negate and deny homosexuality is so powerful and so fundamental that it demands that lesbians and gay men *prove* their self-identification by acting out their desires (Trenchard, 1989; Sister Marla, 1985). Furthermore, the imperative of identifying and labelling 'perverse' sexual minorities gives rise to the association of particular sexual acts with lesbian and gay sexuality. Thus the practice of anal intercourse has been assigned a key definitive status in the construction of gay male sexuality within heterosexual discourse, and has been accepted as such, often in recalcitrant celebration, by some gay men (Patton, 1990a). A parallel process has privileged cunnilingus as definitive, indeed, some have argued, 'symptomatic' of lesbianism. (One psychoanalytic theory of the aetiology of lesbianism (cited by Klaich, 1989) suggests that women who have not outgrown their longing for the breast turn to the clitoris as a substitute nipple; why we should prefer the clitoris to a mouthful of penis, or, indeed, to the actual nipple of a woman lover, is not addressed.)

This discursive structuration of sexual identities around specific sexual practices is clearly problematic for safer sex promotion. Defining anal intercourse as a gay practice reinforces oppressive cultural stereotypes and neglects the needs of those gay men who do not enjoy anal intercourse and of those heterosexual couples who do. Likewise, safer sex advice recommending dental dams and latex gloves to lesbians suggests that cunnilingus and finger-fucking somehow 'belong' to lesbian sex, and are not important to heterosexuals. Significantly, both pornography and safer sex information overtly privilege penis-in-vagina penetration, potentially a high-risk activity for HIV transmission, as central to heterosex (Richardson, 1990; Jackson, 1988; Jeffreys, 1990), an observation which should make us cynical with regard to any claims for the radicalism of either.

Sexual Risk

The notion of risk is profoundly gendered. For some men, an element of risk apparently makes sex more exciting (Jeffreys, 1987; Patton, 1985), a fact which introduces a certain element of farce into HIV/AIDS health promotion. For women, the association of risk and sex is ancient (English Collective of Prostitutes, 1988; Chapman, 1988; Richardson, 1990). Rape, sexual abuse, and pregnancy are risks. Cervical cancer is a risk. The most recent statistics for the UK show that in 1989 there were 4,496 women known to have cervical cancer, of whom 2,170 died (Women's National Cancer Control Campaign, personal communication). In the same year there were 848 people known to have AIDS, of whom 301 died (CDSC Monthly Report, 1990). There is no 'buddying service' for women with cervical cancer, no affirmative counselling; more importantly, there has never been a campaign to promote the kinds of safer sex which might well have prevented their deaths.

Sexual Pleasure

The liberal rhetoric of gay liberation unproblematically elides sexual pleasure with freedom, with political radicalism, indeed with life itself (Watney, 1987; Bronski, 1989). As early as 1979, feminists were mocking the liberal male assertion that 'sex, more sex, and sex the powers didn't like would bring the house down' (Lederer, 1979). In the context of AIDS, there is an insistence that safer sex must be pleasurable, and must be seen to be pleasurable, because 'If sex were not pleasurable people would not be at risk' (Watney, 1987). Whose pleasure is assumed here? Decades of feminist research have shown that the notion of sexual pleasure is a profoundly problematic one for women. The most recent studies show that women, on the whole, derive little pleasure from heterosexual sex (Gavey, 1987, 1989, 1993; Holland *et al.*, 1990; Hite, 1987), that they are not able to ask for what they want (Gavey, 1987; Hite, 1987), that their pleasure is *not* taken into account in their relationships, that they are, in fact, utterly disempowered, silenced, ignored, and often engaging in sexual activity in conditions of fear and physical discomfort. One of the young Australian women interviewed by Nicola Gavey vividly describes the particular paralysis which removes women's control over their own bodies during sexual encounters with men, 'if someone was standing on my foot I'd fucking tell her . . . Someone's got their penis in my vagina . . . and I don't feel able to ask them to stop. It's just *ridiculous'* (Gavey, 1990). It is tempting to argue that if sex were not pleasurable to men, women would not be at risk. Sexual pleasure, then, being both fundamentally gendered and inequitably assigned, is hardly a straightforward concept on which to base the promotion of safer sex.

Representation

Consideration of sexual pleasure, and of the problematic nature of women's sexual pleasure in particular, leads us back to the question of the representative practices of pornography and safer sex materials. There is a simplistic argument which states that 'Pornography can't be sick because sexuality isn't sick. The pornographic sickness doesn't reside in the works of pornography, but in the minds of erotophobes' (Witomski, 1985, cited in Watney, 1987). It is this familiar elision which would have it that using pornographic imagery is the only effective way to promote safer sex. I would argue that the elision of sex and pornography in this way is in fact profoundly problematic in the context of HIV/AIDS health promotion. 'Sex is always historically and socially specific, and its meaning is a site of constant struggle' writes Foucault (1978). Pornography, and indeed safer sex propaganda, are not transparent practices, reflecting a pre-existing sexual 'reality' elsewhere constructed. They are signifying practices, 'discourses through which material power is exercised, and through which the gendered relations of power which inhere in sex are reflected, re-established and perpetuated' (Gavey, 1989, 1990). Moreover, to elide pornographic representation with sexual pleasure is to ignore the 'importance of language/representation as a *constitutive* process' (Gavey, 1990). The social discourses available to men and women constitute our subjectivities and reproduce or challenge existing gender relations. Pornography is one such social discourse. 'The pornographers', writes Sheila Jeffreys (1987), 'are involved in the construction of sexuality'. Safer sex promotional material is, of course, another such constitutive discourse. In the context of homophobia, AIDS commentary has developed a well-theorized understanding of how this process operates, and how essential an awareness of it is in work around HIV/AIDS. Watney (1987) writes: 'The ways in which gay men are able to organise in relation to AIDS . . . is (sic) dependent on our image of ourselves, and this imagery is always and everywhere subject to state intervention and control'. If the social discourses of gay male sexuality directly affect the way in which gay men are able to respond to AIDS, and I think this quite clearly is so, the same is true of everybody else. What social discourses are available to women to support our response to AIDS?

Nicola Gavey (1990) argues that 'in dominant discourses on hetero-sexuality women are positioned as passive subjects who are encouraged to comply with sex with men irrespective of their own desire'. Janet Holland and her colleagues discovered that the young women they interviewed actually defined 'sex' as being focused on male pleasure, a finding which powerfully confirms the *constitutive* nature of such discourses. A feminist interrogation of medical texts, such as that undertaken by Scully and Bart, reveals such gems as this: 'an important feature of sex desire in the man is the urge to dominate the woman and subjugate her to his will: in the woman acquiescence to the masterful takes a high place'. Clearly, the social discourses available to women constitute a sexual subjectivity, an experience of desire, which is not merely responsive and passive, but negative. Female desire is simply not permissible, not imaginable, not there. Dale Spender (1985) echoes Dorothy Hage in noting that 'there is no term for normal sexual power in women'.

A feminist/Foucauldian analysis of femininity begins to suggest the ways in which dominant discourses of femininity construct the female body as the paradigmatic site for establishing and perpetuating gendered relations of power. Woman, writes Sandra Lee Bartky, is 'a self-policing subject, a self committed to a relentless self-surveillance. This self-surveillance is a form of obedience to patriarchy. It is also a reflection in the woman's consciousness that *she* is under surveillance in a way that *he* is not, that whatever she may become, she is importantly a body designed to please or excite' (Bartky, 1988). Or as John Berger put it, 'Women are there to feed an appetite, not to have any of their own' (Berger, 1972).

This discursive positioning of woman as the object of desire, 'innocent' of sexual agency, has far-reaching implications for the sex-uality of both men and women, whether heterosexual, lesbian or gay. (It is merely disingenuous to suggest that lesbians and gay men are somehow outside the realm of discourse.) Catharine Stimpson points out that this image of women as *innocent,* especially of sexual desire, makes logically necessary the image of women as *victims* in pornography. If desire is unavailable to women, then sex can only be something done by men to women. If autonomous sexual pleasure is unavailable to women, then sexual practices which foreground male pleasure are inevitable. This insight into the vicious circle of the discursive structuration of femininity has profound and disturbing implications for HIV/AIDS health promotion.

It has long been clear that heterosexual women stand to gain much from non-penetrative sex. AIDS has not changed that, it has simply added to the urgency. Safer sex demands that we de-emphasize penetration. Safer sex also demands that partners negotiate sexual practice. Yet it is clear that both demands are quite simply impossible within the context of a heteropatriarchal discourse which constructs sex as penetration of a woman by a man, privileging male sexual pleasure and constructing female subjectivity as powerless, pleasureless and androcentric (Wilton and Aggleton, 1990). Central to the successful promotion of safer sex are the feminist challenge to these powerful social scripts and the feminist demand for the recognition of autonomous female sexuality. To succeed in controlling this epidemic demands nothing less than a radical rupture of the discursive processes which shape female and male sexual subjectivity and which differentially assign power to men and women.

Pornography and Safer Sex

So what does feminism, in particular the feminist critique of pornography, have to offer HIV/AIDS health promotion? American Moral Majority representative Victor Cline believes that 'pornography leads to multiple partners which, if conditions are right, may lead to AIDS' (Watney, 1987). Quite clearly, this kind of nonsense must be challenged. Nor is it appropriate to call for censorship in response to pornography (Dworkin, 1988, MacKinnon, 1989). Feminist activists are only too well aware that censorship is far more likely to be used against socially marginalized groups such as lesbians than against *Mayfair* or *Playboy* (Kelly, 1990; Young, 1989; Cole, 1989). Equally, the elision of sex, pornography and life is both foolish and counterproductive. Crucially, it ignores power. Power, as Foucault somewhat unfortunately puts it, 'penetrates and controls every pleasure' (Bartky, 1988). Power, as feminist Chris Weedon (1987) puts it, 'inheres in difference, and is a dynamic of control and lack of control between discourses and the subjects, constituted by discourses, who are their agents'. Power does not inhere equally in masculinity and femininity. For gay men there may be 'a simple distinction between consensual and coercive forms of sex' (Watney, 1987). For women there is no such simple distinction. Women 'live in the world pornography creates' (MacKinnon, 1989). In such a context, sexual explicitness cannot be, per se, radical. Indeed, it risks becoming, in Gunter Schmidt's words, a 'pillar of the establishment' (Schmidt, 1990). In order to be politically radical, and in order to be effective, safer sex materials have to challenge, rather than reproduce, those discursive practices which disempower women. We have not yet even begun to develop such a radical discourse around safer sex. Safer sex promotion, which Bea Campbell (1987) dismisses as 'penetration propaganda', has so far resoundingly upheld the sexual status quo.

Simon Watney writes of 'the urgent, the desperate need to eroticize information about safer sex', and warns that if this is not done, 'tens of thousands of more lives (sic) (will be) cruelly sacrificed on the twin altars of prudery and homophobia' (Watney, 1987). The task of 'eroticizing safer sex' is just not that simple, nor is it one we should undertake without recognizing our responsibility to challenge, rather than to collude with, the unequal social relations of power which are implicit in every sexual act, every sexualized text or image, and which act so powerfully to impede the practice of safer sex. To resist the erotophobic construction of AIDS as the consequences of perversion is undoubtedly an urgent task. Yet to call pornography to the service of safer sex is merely to collude with oppression in the name of libertarianism, and to fail utterly to engage with the core issue of power. What is needed is the development of a representational practice which challenges the dominant discursive construction of gender and of sexuality, and which creates a space for desire, male as well as female. ' The question for pornography', writes Catharine MacKinnon, 'is what eroticism *is* as distinct from the subordination of women' (MacKinnon, 1989). That is a question which we must demand of safer sex promotional practice if HIV/AIDS prevention is to work.

Notes

1   Throughout this chapter, I shall use AIDS (rather than HIV or HIV/AIDS) to refer to the social construction of AIDS which sees it as a medical, moral and metaphorical 'disease'.

References

ALLISON, DOROTHY (1984) 'Public Silence, Private Terror', in VANCE, CAROLE (Ed.) *Pleasure and Danger: Exploring Female Sexuality*, London, Pandora.

BARTKY, SANDRA LEE (1988) 'Foucault, Femininity and the Modernization of Patriarchal Power', in DIAMOND, IRENE and QUINBY, LEE (Eds) *Feminism and Foucault: Reflections on Resistance* Boston, Northeastern University Press, pp. 61–86.

BERGER, JOHN (1972) *Ways of Seeing*, Harmondsworth, Penguin.

BRONSKI, MICHAEL (1989) 'Death and the Erotic Imagination', in CARTER, ERICA and WATNEY, SIMON (Eds) *Taking Liberties: AIDS and Cultural Politics*, London, Serpent's Tail.

BROWNMILLER, SUSAN (1975) *Against Our Will: Men, Women and Rape*, New York, Simon and Schuster.

CAMPBELL, BEA (1987) 'Bealine' *Marxism Today*, December, p. 9

CHAPMAN, KAREN (1988) 'Safer Sex for Some', *Lib Ed*, Summer, pp. 4–6.

COLE, SUSAN G. (1989) *Pornography and the Sex Crisis*, Toronto, Amanita.

DAVIES, KATH; DICKEY, JULIENNE and STRATFORD, TERESA (Eds) (1987) *Out of Focus: Writings on Women and the Media*, London, The Women's Press.

DOWSETT, GARY (1991) Keynote address given at the Fifth Social Aspects of AIDS Conference, London, 23 March.

DWORKIN, ANDREA (1988) *Letters from a War Zone*, London, Secker and Warburg.

ELLIS, KATE; O'DAIR, BARBARA and TALLMER, ABBY (1990) 'Feminism and Pornography', *Feminist Review*, no. 36, pp. 15–17.

ENGLISH COLLECTIVE OF PROSTITUTES (1988) *Prostitute Women and AIDS: Resisting the Virus of Repression*, London, English Collective of Prostitutes.

FOUCAULT, MICHAEL (1978) *The History of Sexuality: Volume 1: An Introduction*, Harmondsworth, Penguin.

FRUTCHEY, CHUCK (1990) 'The Role of Community-Based Organisations in AIDS and STD Prevetion', in PAALMAN, MARIA (Ed.) *Promoting Safer Sex*, Amsterdam, Swets and Zeitlinger.

GAVEY, NICOLA (1989) 'Feminist Poststructuralism and Discourse Analysis', *Psychology of Women Quarterly*, no. 13, pp. 459–75.

GAVEY, NICOLA (1990) *Technologies and Effects of Heterosexual Subjugation*, Department of Psychology, University of Auckland.

GAVEY, NICOLA (1993) 'Technologies of Heterosexual Subjugation', in WILKINSON, S. and KITZINGER, C. (Eds) *Heterosexuality*, Feminism and Psychology Special Issue.

HITE, SHERE (1987) *Women and Love: A Cultural Revolution in Progress*, Harmondsworth, Penguin.

HOLLAND, JANET; RAMAZANOGLU, CAROLINE; SCOTT, SUE; SHARPE, SUE and THOMSON, RACHEL (1990) 'Don't Die of Ignorance — I Nearly Died of Embarrassment: Condoms in Context' in WRAP Paper 2, London, Tufnell.

HOLLWAY, WENDY (1984) 'Women's Power in Heterosexual Sex', *Women's Studies International Forum*, no. 7, pp. 63–8.

HOMANS, HILARY and AGGLETON, PETER (1988) 'Health Education, HIV Infection and AIDS', in AGGLETON, PETER and HOMANS, HILARY (Eds) *Social Aspects of AIDS*, Lewes, Falmer Press.

JACKSON, GAIL (1988) 'Promotion of Safer Sex or the Patriarchy, Misogyny and the Condom', unpublished paper.

JEFFREYS, SHEILA (1987) 'The Body Politic — The Campaign Against Pornography', in DAVIES, KATH; DICKEY, JULIENNE and STRATFORD, TERESA (Eds) *Out of Focus: Writings on Women and the Media*, London, The Women's Press.

JEFFREYS, SHEILA (1990) *Anticlimax: A Feminist Perspective on the Sexual Revolution*, London, The Women's Press.

KAVENEY, ROZ (1990) 'She's Got to Have It', *Square Peg*, no. 27, p. 17.

KELLY, LIZ (1990) 'Abuse in the Making', *Trouble and Strife*, no. 19, Summer, pp. 32–7.

KLAICH, D. (1989) *Woman Plus Woman* (2nd edn.) Tallahassee, Naiad Press.

LEDERER, LAURA (1979) 'Introduction', in LEDERER, LAURA (Ed.) *Take Back the Night*, London, The Women's Press.

McGRATH, ROBERTA (1990) 'Dangerous Liaisons: Health, Disease and Representation', in BOFFIN, TESSA and GUPTA, SUNIL (Eds) *Ecstatic Antibodies: Resisting the AIDS Mythology*, London, Rivers Oram.

MACKINNON, CATHARINE A. (1989) 'Pornography: Not a Moral Issue', in KLEIN, RENATE D. and STEINBERG, DEBORAH LYNN (Eds) *Radical Voices: A Decade of Resistance from* Women's Studies International Forum, Oxford, Pergamon Press.

MANCHESTER CITY COUNCIL HIV/AIDS POLICY GROUP (1990) *AIDS, HIV and Civil Liberties* (Report of Conference which took place 22–23 March 1990).

SISTER MARLA (1985) 'Gay and Celibate at Sixty-Five', in CURB, ROSEMARY and MANAHAN, NANCY (Eds) *Lesbian Nuns: Breaking Silence*, Tallahassee, Naiad Press.

PAALMAN, MARIA (Ed.) (1990) *Promoting Safer Sex*, Amsterdam, Swets and Zeitlinger.

PATTON, CINDY (1985) *Sex and Germs: The Politics of AIDS*, Boston, South End Press.

PATTON, CINDY (1990a) 'Thinking on Your Feet: A CMM Approach to Training Peer Educators', unpublished paper.

PATTON, CINDY (1990b) 'Safer Sex as Resistance to Societal Control and Moralism' paper presented at the First Nordic Conference on Safer Sex, Stockholm, March.

POLLOCK, GRISELDA (1987) 'What's Wrong with Images of Women', in BETTERTON, ROSEMARY (Ed.) *Looking On: Images of Femininity in the Visual Arts and the Media*, London, Pandora.

RICHARDSON, DIANE (1990) 'AIDS Education and Women: Sexual and Reproductive Issues', in AGGLETON, PETER; DAVIES, PETER and HART, GRAHAM (Eds) *AIDS: Individual, Cultural and Policy Dimensions*, London, Falmer Press.

RODGERSON, GILLIAN and SEMPLE, LINDA (1990) 'Who Watches the Watchwomen? Feminists Against Censorship', *Feminist Review*, no. 36, pp. 19–28.

RULE, JANE (1985) *A Hot-Eyed Moderate*, Talahassee, Naiad Press.

SCHMIDT, GUNTER (1990) 'The Influence of AIDS on Sexuality' in PAALMAN, MARIA (Ed.) *Promoting Safer Sex*, Amsterdam, Swets and Zeitlinger.

SCULLY, DIANA and BART, PAULINE (1973) 'A Funny Thing Happened on the Way to the Orifice: Women in Gynaecology Text Books' in HUBER, JOAN (Ed.) *Changing Women in a Changing Society*, University of Chicago Press.

SEATON, JANE (1986) 'Pornography Annoys', in CURRAN, JAMES (Ed.) *Bending Reality: The State of the Media*, London, Pluto.

SEGAL, LYNNE (1990) 'Lessons from the Past: Feminism, Sexual Politics and the Challenge of AIDS', in CARTER, ERICA and WATNEY, SIMON (Eds) *Taking Liberties: AIDS and Cultural Politics*, London, Serpent's Tail.

SPENDER, DALE (1985) *Man Made Language*, 2nd ed., London, Routledge and Kegan Paul.

STIMPSON, CATHARINE R. (1988) *Where the Meanings Are: Feminism and Cultural Spaces*, London, Routledge.

TREICHLER, PAULA (1987) 'AIDS, Homophobia and Biomedical Discourse: An Epidemic of Signification', *October*, no. 43, pp. 32–6.

TRENCHARD, L. (1989) *Being A Lesbian*, London, Gay Men's Press.

TUTTLE, LISA (1986) *Encyclopaedia of Feminism*, London, Arrow Books.

WATNEY, SIMON (1987) *Policing Desire: Pornography, AIDS and the Media*, London, Methuen.

WATNEY, SIMON (1990a) 'Safer Sex as Community Practice', in AGGLETON, PETER; DAVIES, PETER and HART, GRAHAM (Eds) *AIDS: Individual, Cultural and Policy Dimensions*, London, Falmer Press.

WATNEY, SIMON (1990b) 'Representing AIDS', in BOFFIN, TESSA and GUPTA, SUNIL (Eds) *Ecstatic Antibodies: Resisting the AIDS Mythology,* London, Rivers Oram.

WEEDON, CHRIS (1987) *Feminist Practice and Poststructuralist Theory,* Oxford, Basil Blackwell.

WEEKS, JEFFREY (1990) 'Post-modern AIDS?', in BOFFIN, TESSA and GUPTA, SUNIL, (Eds) *Ecstatic Antibodies: Resisting the AIDS Mythology,* London, Rivers Oram.

WILLIAMSON, JUDITH (1987) 'Decoding Advertisements', in BETTERTON, ROSEMARY, (Ed.) *Looking On: Images of Femininity in the Visual Arts and Media,* London, Pandora.

WILTON, TAMSIN (1990a) 'AIDS: Working with the 'Isms", *British Journal of Sociology of Education,* vol. 11, no. 2, pp. 223–38.

WILTON, TAMSIN (1990b) *Not the Same Kind of Difference: Equal Opportunities and Lesbianism, a Feminist Perspective,* University of Bristol, MSc dissertation.

WILTON, TAMSIN (1991) 'Tits and Bums and Saving Lives: HIV/AIDS and the New Politics of Pornography' (under review).

WILTON, TAMSIN (1992) 'Desire and the Politics of Representation: Issues for Lesbians and Heterosexual Women', in HINDS, HILARY; PHOENIX ANN and STACEY, JACKIE (Eds) *Working Out: New Directions for Women's Studies,* London, Falmer Press.

WILTON, TAMSIN and AGGLETON, PETER (1990) *Young People and Safer Sex,* paper given at the First Nordic Conference on Safer Sex, Stockholm, March.

WILTON, TAMSIN and AGGLETON, PETER (1991) 'Condoms, Coercion and Control: Heterosexuality and the Limits to HIV/AIDS Health Education', in AGGLETON, PETER; DAVIES, PETER and HART, GRAHAM (Eds) *AIDS: Responses, Interventions and Care,* London, Falmer Press.

WITOMSKI, T.R. (1985) 'The "Sickness" of Pornography', *New York Native,* no. 121, pp. 11–13.

YOUNG, CRAIG (1989) 'Split Desire: Policing Sado-Masochisms', *Sites: A Journal for Radical Perspectives on Culture,* no. 19, Spring, Dept of Social Anthropology, Massey University, New Zealand, pp. 167–71.

Chapter 6

Visible and Invisible Women in AIDS Discourses

Jenny Kitzinger

Introduction

Woman is white, heterosexual and middle-class. She is everybody's sister, wife, and mother. 'Woman' and the related term 'everyone' have a special place in the mainstream AIDS lexicon. The pure category 'woman', unsullied by any prefix, represents 'the ordinary person' who does not use illegal drugs or engage in promiscuous or homosexual sex. She is a symbol for 'the family', the 'general population' and all the 'innocent victims' of AIDS.

But 'woman' is not the only representation of female existence in the AIDS media coverage. She shares the stage with the prostitute, the nymphomaniac, the evil mother and the 'African woman'. These positive and negative female personae in the AIDS morality tale tell us a great deal both about the representation of the syndrome and about the social construction of female sexuality. This chapter focuses on problematic media representations of Good-Women and Bad-Women and explores how these are mobilized in ways which undermine 'general public' concern about the AIDS epidemic and further stigmatize gay men, lesbians and other 'deviants'.

Method

The findings discussed here draw on the AIDS Media Research Project conducted with my colleagues Peter Beharrell, David Miller and Kevin Williams. The project as a whole involved a study of the production, content and effect of AIDS media messages. The content analysis involved detailed coding of all the main press and television news coverage between November 1988 and April 1990. The 'effect' part of the study involved tape-recorded discussions with fifty-two different groups of people. The sample included both 'general population' and 'special interest' groups — the latter were chosen because they might be expected to have particular perspectives or insights into the issues, either because they had some kind of professional involvement in the field or because they were members of so-called 'high-risk' populations. So, for example, we conducted discussions with a group of women whose children attended the same playgroup and a team of civil engineers working on the same site; but we also ran sessions with prison officers, male prostitutes, IV drug users and lesbians (see table 6.1). In this chapter I will be focusing predominantly on the 'general population' or 'mainstream professional' perspectives rather than documenting the oppositional readings of politicized individuals such as the gay men or lesbian activists. For discussion of oppositional readings see Kitzinger, 1993.

Woman = Heterosexual

One of the ironies of the AIDS media coverage is that it has challenged the linguistic assumption of heterosexuality for men. Its initial prominence as a 'gay plague' means that 'man' is not automatically assumed to mean 'heterosexual man'. The same is not true for the term 'woman'. On the contrary, the media coverage has both illustrated and reinforced heterosexist assumptions about women. HIV/AIDS statistics are routinely presented in ways which distinguish between men of different sexual 'persuasions' but treat women as an amorphous, single category e.g. 'Homosexual and bisexual men accounted for 1,680 cases. Seventy-one women had developed the disease' (*Daily Telegraph,* February 1989). Lesbians are rendered invisible: women are referred to in explicit contrast to 'the homosexual community' and we are urged to use condoms or to avoid bisexuals (suggestions which are, at best, confusing for those of us who choose other women as lovers).

Between November 1988 and April 1990 there were over 2,500 articles about AIDS in the British national and Scottish press. Only five of these stated that sex between women might be safer than heterosexual sex and none included information about safer sex specifically aimed at lesbians. At the same time there were over 500 individual statements about women and the transmission of HIV, but only six statements made it explicit that they were about heterosexual women, and three of these are attributable to the same source — they were in media reports of a conference paper given by Judy Bury (another contributor to this book).

Table 6.1   Groups participating in the study

Group	Number of groups of this type	Total number of participants in these groups
I People with occupational interest, involvement or responsibility		
Doctors	1	4
Nurses/health visitors	1	6
Social workers	1	4
Drug workers	1	5
SACRO* workers	1	3
Police staff	2	16
Prison staff	5	32
Teachers	1	5
Community council workers	1	3
African journalists (Nigeria, Zaire, Zimbabwe, Uganda)	1	4
II People targeted as 'high-risk groups' by the media or with some special knowledge of, or political involvement in, the issue		
Male prostitutes	2	6
Gay men	2	9
Lesbians	2	6
Family of a gay man	1	4
Prisoners	5	28
Clients of NACRO and SACRO*	4	27
Clients in drug rehabilitation centre	1	7
Young people in intermediate treatment	1	5
III People who, as a group, have no obvious special interest or involvement in the issue		
Retired people	3	25
Women living on the same Glasgow estate	1	4
School students	3	26
Women with children attending playgroup	2	14
Engineers	2	18
Round Table group	1	14
American students	1	25
Janitors	1	7
Market researchers	1	3
Cleaners	1	4
British college students (England, Scotland and Wales)	3	37
Total number of all groups	52	
Total number of participants in all groups		351

Note: * These acronyms stand for the Scottish and the National Associations for the Care and Resettlement of Offenders.

Given dominant heterosexist assumptions about 'woman' and the marginalization of lesbians, it is not surprising that 'woman' is also used as the symbol of normality in the AIDS saga. Within the mainstream AIDS coverage she has become a rare female personification of Joe Bloggs (a part less easily played by a man because of the association of AIDS with male homosexuality — and heaven forbid that a gay man might represent 'the man in the street'!). When asked to write a news bulletin caption using a photograph of a white woman holding a child, several of the audience groups used this picture to illustrate statements about 'society at large', 'normal, everyday people' and 'the general population'.

More specifically, 'woman' also represents the nuclear family. 'AIDS is claiming the lives of so many women and children that', we are told, it is now 'a family disease' (*Scotsman*, 23 November 1989) — as if gay men and drug users cannot be considered part of 'real families' at all — as if they are nobody's father, brother, husband or son. The institution of The Family as it is represented here does not contain deviants, it is only threatened by them. Deviants endanger 'family values', betray their parents and undermine the stability of the nuclear unit — a perspective graphically illustrated by some of the government anti-drug posters. One identified a series of needle marks in a user's arm as 'hits' paid for by stealing various items from his brother and parents: 'Kevin's pocket-money', 'Dad's wallet' and 'Mum's housekeeping'. Another advert showed someone holding some smack with the telling caption: 'This is the last of his mum's wedding ring' (see Clark, 1988).

Woman, as wife and mother, also serves to personify the 'innocent victims' of AIDS. We are invited to sympathize with 'Agony of innocent mum' and to be horrified that 'curse hits ordinary families' (*Sun*, 22 February 1990; *Star*, 29 August 1989). *The Times* (30 September 1989) proclaimed that 'The saddest stories are from women living conventional lives who did not know, or did not want to know, the truth about their partner's bisexuality, or past history of drug-taking'. The *Sun* treats us to the headline: 'My husband was a hotshot lawyer who slunk off for long walks alone — and came home to me with AIDS'. Male homosexuality is portrayed as an alien and 'beastly' threat: 'for when night fell, he slunk off to the homosexual bath houses in the seedier parts of Manhattan's Greenwich Village. Using a false name and with an anorak hood pulled over his face the $100,000-a-year lawyer picked up "rough trade" sex' (*Sun*, 2 March 1990).

This construction of 'woman' as a symbol of all that is threatened by deviance was closely echoed by some of the audience groups. One research participant described women as 'innocent bystanders' (as if they were the accidental victims of terrorist activity) and another talked about bisexual men as 'no better than murderers'.

In theory, however, 'woman' as emblem of 'cleanliness', 'community' and 'caring' should be able to extend those qualities to 'the AIDS problem'. Princess Diana, in particular, might have been expected to achieve this through her high-profile concern about the epidemic. Ironically, however, the media often reported her involvement in this issue in terms which imply some danger. They describe her 'courage' and 'devotion' as if there really were some risk of 'contagion'. As the media dances attendance on Diana as 'The Caring Princess' they also often ignore the gruelling, unglamorous, and poverty-stricken task of day-to-day caring carried out by women all over the world — where caring means hard physical labour as well as emotional exhaustion. While Princess Diana's actions have certainly done a great deal to challenge notions of casual transmission ('They wouldn't let her shake hands with them if you could catch it that way') they seem to have done little to alter people's basic views on AIDS. In particular many research participants expressed admiration for her work but, at the same time, continued to discriminate against 'guilty victims' of the virus.

In fact, when Princess Diana's actions appeared to challenge the innocent/guilty division — for instance in, literally, embracing gay men — sections of the press (even the usually loyal and royalist newspapers) employed the language and imagery of sexism against her. The *Sun,* dismissing Diana as 'the royal clothes horse', declared that she seemed to 'have a fascination with terminal illness' and suggested: 'maybe Prince Charles should buy her a stethoscope for Christmas, he might get to play doctors and nurses' (*Sun,* 4 December 1989). The *Star,* alarmed that she was not confining her attention to innocent babies, suggested that it was 'about time her husband put down his royal foot and told Princess Diana "No more visits to adult AIDS centres"' (*Star,* 1 August 1990). The *Evening Standard* even suggested that her commitment to people with AIDS was symptomatic of a common female mental disorder — 'co-dependency' — and compared her to 'the saintly wife who sticks by her alcoholic husband year after relapsing year' and 'the loyal secretary who never forgets the boss's wife's birthday' (*Evening Standard,* 8 October 1991). Evidently, even royalty can be 'put in their place' as women. (For discussion of tabloid press ambivalence about Princess Diana, see Beharrell, 1993.)

Princess Diana is only one manifestation of the woman 'embracing' the AIDS crisis. In various fictional dramatizations of the 'AIDS story', white, middle-class, 'ordinary' women have been featured in this position, in relation to their own families. In these dramas the wife/mother character serves to model attempts by the humane family unit to 'come to terms with' deviant offspring. She acts as the representative of liberal morality — articulating ignorance but ultimately able to 'move on' and accept what has happened. As such she is supposed to provide a point of identification for the 'ordinary viewer' and a bridge to a more 'enlightened' understanding. This was clearly the intention behind many of the AIDS dramas such as *Our Sons, An Early Frost* and *Sweet As You Are*.

Our Sons and *An Early Frost* both told the story of gay men with AIDS but each focused on the reactions of the men's blood relatives. Such dramas clearly challenged the exclusion of gay men from popular conceptions of The Family. However, the primary focus on the biological family also served to 'neuter' the topic and rip it out of context — presenting the viewer with gay men shorn of their sexual identity. As Treichler points out, even the title of *Our Sons* 'contains its volatile topic within familial bonds' and the programme 'offers viewers the family's perspectives, treats homosexuality as a central — and legitimate — problem for the straight characters, makes little reference to AIDS as a national health care crisis, and perhaps, above all, renders the rage and political mobilisation of activist groups invisible, indeed incomprehensible' (Treichler, in press). These dramas ignore gay men's commitment to each other in the face of AIDS and implicitly dismiss the passionate networks of support and friendship within the gay communities as 'pretended family relations'. The focus is shifted away from the impact of AIDS on entire communities or even on the infected individual himself. 'We see how AIDS affects a young man's mother, father, sister, brother-in-law and grandmother. There is no consideration given to the fact that this is happening to him — not them' (Russo, quoted in Treichler, in press).

These reservations about the structure of such dramas were borne out by our empirical work with the 'general population' and 'mainstream professional' audience groups. They remembered these programmes as 'family dramas' and recalled the reactions of the men's mothers in particular. Many of the research participants could identify with a mother's position, but the very fact that the story concerns a woman's attempts to come to terms with AIDS *within her own family* limited the transformatory impact of the tale. Mothers, they said, could excuse anything. One group, for example, recalled a TV discussion with a woman whose son had killed himself rather than admit that he was gay. This group were particularly hostile to homosexuality but recalled this mother's statement that 'she would rather see her boy a happy homosexual than an unhappy not-homosexual'. 'Ah, well', replied another member of the group 'you see, *that's* mother-love' (Retired people,

Group 2). Many people seemed to believe that a woman must support her own 'flesh and blood' but saw this as an indiscriminate maternal duty without general moral or political content. A mother would support her son if he had AIDS, just as she would if he turned out to be a rapist: 'you would support them, no matter what (. . .) you may not like what they have done or whatever but I think you have still got that support for them — a *mother* does anyway' (Cleaners). A woman's change of heart because of her son's seropositive status was not then recognized as offering a wider example to the 'general population'.

Other AIDS dramas have focused on cases of heterosexual AIDS, again within a family context. *'Sweet As You Are'* concerned a male lecturer who discovered that he was HIV-positive after an affair with a female student. A great deal of attention was focused on the reactions of his wife. The power of this representation for 'ordinary people' was amply demonstrated by some research participants who praised it for being 'a tale of everyday folk' and 'showing *family* situations with *real people*' (Students, Group 2, emphasis added). As one social worker commented:

I remember that coming home to me (. . .) I suppose it was very much *the human element,* sort of *families,* you know, *children* and . . . it could be anyone (. . .) it suddenly comes home that, you know, it is not just gay people, it's not just coloured people, but it's actually anybody in this room that could be infected. (Social workers, emphasis added).

The irony of using the figure of a white, middle-class woman to 'bring home' such messages is that it exploits and reinforces dominant understandings about whose life 'counts'. Such dramatizations do not reflect the real demographic distribution of HIV infection and do nothing to challenge underlying views about what constitutes 'the human element'. Nor do they counteract assumptions about the type of people who make up 'real people' or 'everyday folk'. The social worker's last sentence revealed her own (incorrect) assumption that 'anybody in this room' did not include gay people — at least one lesbian was present.

The figure of Good-Woman, then, within mainstream AIDS discourses, is deeply problematic. 'Woman' excludes large proportions of the female population and her 'ordinariness' and 'innocence' is used as a foil against which to judge 'the deviants'. Even when Good-Woman engages with the AIDS crisis (as a princess or a mother) her 'compassion' is excused or dismissed as a feminine/maternal trait which has no wider political implication.

The figure of Bad-Woman is equally stereotyped and destructive. In contrast to the innocent 'whiter-than-white' middle-class woman (pillar of the family, emblem of heterosexual respectability, symbol of hearth and home) Bad-Woman appears as dark temptress, vamp, prostitute and 'AIDS carrier'. The extent to which journalists and members of 'the general population' may empathize with the former manifestation of womanhood is equalled by the force with which they condemn the latter. The division of women into good and bad pivots on polarities such as home/street, controlled/loose, day/night, light/dark. 'Streetwalkers', 'loose women' and 'ladies of the night' are the mirror opposites of the 'housewife'. As feminists have pointed out, both the condemnation of Bad-Woman and the equal but opposite adulation of Good-Woman serve to control female sexuality and police the boundaries of acceptability (Morgan, 1970; Rhodes and McNeill, 1985; Smart and Smart, 1978).

Within mainstream AIDS discourse, the reproductive potential of Bad-Woman is transformed into the power to bequeath death to her offspring.[1] Although the 'innocent mother', infected by a blood transfusion or by her husband, may pass on HIV to her children 'through no fault of her own' (*Daily Mirror,* 28 December 1988), other HIV-positive mothers are portrayed as little better than child-murderers. Some research participants talked about the 'crime' of 'babies being subjected to the virus in the womb due to promiscuity and drug-using mothers' and expressed disgust at women who 'give AIDS' to their children: 'you think "you selfish git, look at that", . . .there's a young life ruined due to your stupidity' (Prison staff, Groups 2 and 4). One man suggested that women should be sent to prison if they know they have the virus but still 'go and get themselves pregnant'. Another declared that even more drastic steps were needed: 'drug addicts and prostitutes should be given an operation so they can't have kids' (Janitors).

There was also the suggestion by some white research participants that black women's 'breeding' abilities were directly implicated in the spread of HIV. Black motherhood in Africa was presented as 'indiscriminate': 'their first object in life is to get pregnant (. . .) and they don't mind how many male partners they have, a woman will have children by about five different partners' (Retired people, Group 3) and one young man produced the statement that: 'AIDS originated in Africa, it spread quickly because of the large families. Immigrants brought the condition over' (School students, Group 2).

The promiscuous black woman is presented as a danger to white society as well as her children. She, along with her white counterpart, is also a threat to 'ordinary' heterosexual men. Prostitutes (both black and white) are widely represented as 'reservoirs of infection' and became a familiar sight in AIDS documentaries and news reports. 'Streetwalkers' were filmed, literally, from the male viewpoint of a cruising car, with a male doctor's voice-over detailing how many men one prostitute could infect in a year (see Clark, 1988). It is prostitutes, not their clients, who are identified as the carrier of disease who 'gamble with the lives of others' (*Evening Times,* 1 December 1988). The 'loose' woman, like the gay or bisexual man, is not part of 'the community', she is a vector *through* which disease many infiltrate 'wider society'.[2]

Such images of Bad-Woman as threat are not confined to the mass media, and are certainly not a new phenomenon. The female body has traditionally personified sexual danger. The propaganda against venereal disease during the first and second world wars, for example, focused on *women,* rather than men, as the source of infection. One poster displayed a wholesome-looking young white woman with the slogan: 'She may look clean but pick-ups, good time girls, prostitutes spread syphilis and gonorrhoea'. Another poster showed a prostitute arm-in-arm with Hitler and Hirohito, with the captain 'VD: The Worst of These' (Brandt, 1985). Some of the AIDS health education advertisements of the 1980s and 1990s seemed to repeat this history. Two particularly notorious advertisements showed traditionally attractive, predatory women. The first, a television advertisement, was set in the rather elegant home of a seductive woman who invites a man to stay the night. The advertisement uses traditional cinematic techniques encapsulating the male gaze: 'close-ups of parts of the woman's body alternate with close-ups of his observing eye. The man's face is not seen until the final shot, creating a space into which the viewer/voyeur is invited to insert himself' (Rhodes and Shaughnessy, 1990, p. 58).[3]

The magazine or newspaper equivalent presented the viewer with another traditionally alluring image of womanhood, with the caption: 'If this woman had the virus which leads to AIDS in a few years she could look like the person over the page'. The caption set up the expectation that, on turning the page, one would be confronted by a grisly image of the woman — gaunt and hollow-eyed, a shadow of her former self. However, the following page showed an identical picture with a new caption: 'worrying isn't it'.

That rhetorical question (which lacks a question mark) is targeted in a very specific way. Presumably it is not worrying for anyone with HIV to learn that they will remain lovely and healthy for years to come. However, it *is* worrying for the presumed HIV-negative man who fears being seduced by such a woman. The female figure here, then, is a literal *'Fèmme Fàtale'.* As McGrath writes:

the beautiful face, the long hair, the jumper which falls off the shoulder are all signs of woman as a lure, as a seductress who is out to attract men (an old theme). The advert makes us aware that she is (possibly) the dangerous harbourer not only of disease, but of certain death. Beauty can be a mask that conceals all that is rotten. (McGrath, 1990, p. 147)

The same point is made by a male journalist in presenting his reactions to the advert:

The woman with her perfect features, off-the-shoulder top and inviting red lips, excites me and then — when I turn the page to the identical second picture — frightens me. I've got the message. The thing I most desire could destroy me. Fatal attraction. (*Scotsman*, 14 February 1989).[4]

This mixture of fear and fascination was articulated by several male research participants and some suggested that women with HIV might deliberately set out to infect men. The spectre of the 'vengeful AIDS carrier' is not a uniquely female image (see Kitzinger, 1993) but includes female representatives such as the woman in the archetypal urban myth who seduces a man and then disappears leaving a message scrawled on the mirror in bright red lipstick: 'Welcome to the AIDS club'.

The media have publicized several versions of this story, often trawled from all over the world. There was the woman in Belgrade who 'owned up to bedding FIFTEEN of her colleagues. The pretty victim kept quiet about her illness as she moved from man to man' (*Sun*, 9 March 1989: emphasis in original). There was the prostitute who has the 'killer disease' but 'still regularly plies her trade on the streets' (*Daily Star*, 21 April 1990); and the *Guardian* advertised a forthcoming article with the enticing blurb: 'I have Aids. No one knows it. I go to clubs more now so I can meet new men . . . I've slept with 48 men so far, some of them married. I feel if I have to die of a horrible disease, I won't go alone' (*Guardian*, 29 October 1991).

Such articles evidently captured the imagination of many research participants. They swapped tales of the experiences of 'friends of friends' and told stories that closely echoed media accounts: 'there was a girl, and she actually went out and pulled about half a dozen blokes in a day and just went to bed with them and afterwards said "Guess what, you've got it"' (Prison staff, Group 5).

These men's fears of seductive vengeful women were often tied in with expressions of their own vulnerability to 'sexual urges': 'your willie takes charge, doesn't it'; 'a standing penis has no conscience' (Prison staff, Group 4). Some male research participants even referred to cartoon books to convey (and justify) this experience: 'It's like the wee book "Willie" — you see the guy talking to the wee thingamy, it's got a voice, and all that, it's got a mind of its own. If that reacts you do something about it, don't you?' (Prisoners, Group 3). They repeatedly stated that even if they were concerned about HIV they could not resist sexual invitations from attractive women. As one man said: 'If you go to a dance on a Saturday night (. . .) and a woman comes up and goes: "Listen, I want to go home with you tonight", you're not going to go, like, "Ah, you might have AIDS!". You're going to go, man, *no matter what*' (Prisoners, Group 4). In fact, commenting on the health education advertisement, one prison officer stated: 'I mean, the way that girl looked, who was going to say "sorry darling but I'm not coming back to your place tonight"?' (Prison staff, Group 4).

This sense of their own susceptibility to seduction seemed to fuel their anger against 'AIDS carriers' and was often combined with the assertion that people with HIV should be identified and isolated (presumably partly to protect men from falling foul of temptation). It also included an explicit focus on controlling 'their women'. When asked what he thought we should tell children about AIDS, one young man focused exclusively on daughters and replied: 'I'd go and buy a chastity belt (. . .) so nobody could get at her' (SACRO clients, Group 1).

For themselves 'safer sex' seemed often to mean simply staying away from the 'wrong kind of woman'. Heterosexual male research participants spoke of the need to avoid women with 'stinking holes', 'tarts', 'slags', 'gang-bang Joans', 'dirty nails', 'mattress-backs', 'bits of fluff' and girls with 'a reputation' (Young people in intermediate treatment; SACRO clients; Prisoners, Group 4; Round Table group; School students, Group 2). Some of the white men made explicit reference to the dangers of black women, 'dusky maidens' or 'darkies' who were seen as exotic and 'other' as well as being sexually uncontrolled and immoral (Prisoners, Group 4; SACRO clients, Group 1).[5] The category of women to be avoided at all costs also included women who simply dared to carry or use condoms. One man commented that, if a woman suggested safer sex, then 'I'd want to see them in the light' (Prisoners, Group 4). Another stated that a woman would not present a man with a condom or help him to put it on 'unless she was a dirty nymphy or something — a bird wouldn't do that' (Prisoners, Group 1). Many female members of the groups were well aware of this attitude and in subsequent interviews with young women it was clear that this could inhibit them from insisting on condom use. You don't want to carry condoms, they said, because men will think you are 'easy' and treat you with less respect. One young woman who did get as far as carrying a packet of condoms left them in her bag while she had sex with a man she had only just met — so that he wouldn't think she was a slag — just that she had been overwhelmed by the passion of the moment and was half asleep anyway![6]

There was little acknowledgment from any of the heterosexual men that they themselves might be HIV-positive, and pose a threat to women rather than vice versa. However, one prison officer did recall that the video shown to prison staff implied that it was easier for the virus to pass from male to female than vice versa — a fact that made him think that men might resist condom use because 'maybe you're venting your feelings out on the female because they're more likely to get it from you in a sense than you are going to get it from them' (Prison staff, Group 2).

Conclusions

Sexism, combined with other institutional oppressions such as heterosexism and racism, is a central dynamic in many media representations (including some health education adverts) and popular understandings of AIDS. It has a direct impact on men's and women's perceptions of who might be dangerous and how they might ensure their own safety.

Within the mainstream AIDS discourse, 'women' is employed as a homogeneous and exclusive category which symbolically annihilates lesbians and which precludes the possibility of exploring issues such as what could constitute safer sex (e.g. without penetration) or how to develop a global perspective on AIDS. Female imagery is used to set a conservative moral agenda where 'woman' represents innocence and sexual purity against homosexuals, drug users and 'bad women'. Even when 'ordinary' wives and mothers are used as objects of identification and empathy, as in some TV dramas, this does not breach the boundaries of 'family concern' and fails to create a critique of the AIDS issue within a wider political framework.

Some education initiatives exploit, rather than challenge, existing fears and hostilities. Such strategies may be 'memorable' and have 'impact' but they can also fuel a backlash against women (especially Bad-Women) and against gay men. Such tactics are also counterproductive in the struggle against HIV. Some people within advertising refuse to recognize this. One advertiser spoke of his resentment against colleagues in the Health Education Authority who were so concerned about 'sexism or offending people with AIDS' that they weakened the thrust of advertisements. He accused these female colleagues of, in his words, trying to '*castrate* the advertising for no good reason' (emphasis added).[7]

Developing imaginative representations and health education strategies that recognize differences and communalities between women, and which confront issues of power, is part of 'setting a feminist agenda'. Alongside challenging the structural oppressions discussed elsewhere in this book, we need a radical 'theatre of images' such as that developed by feminists during the early years of the Women's Liberation Movement, by black women and men fighting against racism, by protesters within the peace movements and by different AIDS activists. This means engaging in the 'politics of representation' and wresting control of the imagery of AIDS (Boffin and Gupta, 1990).

Notes

I would like to acknowledge the financial support of the ESRC (grant ref no A44250006). Thanks also to my colleagues — Peter Beharrell, David Miller and Kevin Williams and the grant holders — Mick Bloor, John Eldridge, Sally Macintyre and Greg Philo.

1 Examining the portrayal of women in North American AIDS documentaries, Juhasz concludes: 'there are two kinds of mothers depicted in (AIDS documentaries); the minority, poor and guilty, single mothers of sick babies and the white, middle-class married mothers of innocent victims'. Juhasz describes an American programme in which the camera showed a close-up shot of two baby black girls and the image of a young Latino boy alone in a hospital bed. These children are portrayed not as 'victims of AIDS' but as victims of their own mothers. The voice-over stated: 'Almost all the hundreds of children born with AIDS are *victims of drug users:* either drug-addicted mothers, or mothers who got the virus from an IV-infected husband or lover' (Juhasz, 1990, p. 35, emphasis in original).

2 Although this chapter focuses on the ways in which media messages are accepted by audiences, there was also a considerable degree of *resistance* to mainstream representations among some groups. As one 'rent boy' commented: 'they blame us all the time, and the prostitutes. But we don't spread it, we just get it' (Male prostitutes, Group 2). Although the more middle-class 'general population' groups often talked about prostitutes as 'outside society' (e.g. 'It worries me that it is going to get into the community at large through the prostitute thing' (Family group)) this was less common in the more working-class groups and in those groups where any of the members knew women who were 'on the game'. There was also some cynicism about the government concern about prostitutes. As one woman declared: 'None of the Health Ministers were going to bother their backsides unless they could be going to be infected. Everybody does it, businessmen, the lowest, the highest, the lot, go to prostitutes, go to brothels. They could be catching it now so they're getting their knickers in a pickle, in case their wives catch them!' (Women with children attending playgroup, Group 1).

Engaging in prostitution because of economic necessity was widely presented as far more acceptable than the alleged promiscuous sexual proclivities of rich women who slept around through choice. One research participant conjured up a sort of

'Lady Chatterley' figure: 'Look at the social pages, they're jumping from partner to partner, it's all them with bags of money. Lady Maitland (*sic*) in the *Sunday Express* she's been married to this one and she's left him after three years and she's been married to this one and she's left him after two years (. . .) they're like bloody dogs in the street' (Retired people, Group 1).

3   In evaluation research conducted by The Planning Partnership this advert was experienced by test audience groups as being most relevant to 'affluent Southerners' and was identified by some viewers as a 'London Yuppie' scene (The Planning Partnership, 1988; Wellings and Orton, 1988).

4   Ironically these adverts were also criticized in the mainstream press in the context of attacks on the government campaign against 'heterosexual AIDS'. Newspapers without much of a track record for challenging sexist images attached these advertisements for being 'not only dishonest but effectively misogynistic' (*Sunday Telegraph*, 23 July 1989) and 'a libel on half the population (*Mail on Sunday*, 12 February 1989). The *Sunday Telegraph* advised feminists to unite against the advertisement for stirring up 'gynophobia' (*Sunday Telegraph*, 5 February 1989) and even the *Sun* backed 'the feminists' complaints! These representations of the female body became the battleground for the fight over whether or not HIV could be transmitted through 'normal' sex. The advertisements using attractive women were vilified as 'Phoney face of the war on AIDS' (*Daily Mail*, 7 November 1989) or ridiculed for 'peddling the wholly unjustified notion that pretty young women give you AIDS' (*Standard*, 13 September 1989; see also *Sunday Telegraph*, 6 August 1989).

What was notable in this debate was the way in which different ideas about 'woman' were mobilized. Those arguing that heterosexual sex was *not* a danger tended to downplay the 'vampish' qualities of the image — the woman in the picture was simply described as 'young' and 'pretty' or 'attractive'. The statistics were also manipulated to exclude any but the most 'normal' of women (the 'ordinary woman' described in the first part of this chapter). In arguing that HIV was not transmitted by 'heterosexual sex' some people saw fit to exclude from their calculations any woman who had been infected through heterosexual sex with drug users or bisexuals or who became infected outside the UK.

5   Black people in general were sometimes talked about as 'primitive', 'immoral' and 'dirty'   as 'sexual animals' (see Smith, 1983). African women were presented by some white participants as victims of unbridled black male sexuality and cultural 'backwardness': 'they have sex all the time there' (Prisoners, Group 4); 'Black men won't use condoms' (Civil engineers); 'They marry young', 'the men can have as many wives as they like', 'there's a high risk of child prostitution in all these African countries' (Neighbours). For further discussion of media coverage/audience understandings of 'African AIDS' see Kitzinger and Miller, 1992.

6   We found that there were some 'readings' which clearly differed according to the gender of the respondent. For example, women were more likely than men to *disagree* with the health education slogan: 'AIDS: You are as safe as you want to be'. This was sometimes explicitly linked with their own fears of sexual coercion or the belated discovery that a male partner had been unfaithful. However some male research participants, e.g. within the groups of gay men, male prostitutes and male prisoners, expressed similar points of view, challenging the potentially 'victim-blaming' nature of the 'you're as safe as you want to be' message.

7   Some of the representations coming out of the Health Education Authority are a product of conflict between the health educators (who often have a feminist critique) and the advertising staff for whom concern with 'impact' outweighed concern about 'victim blaming, stereotyping and stigmatising' (Miller and Williams, 1993). Some of the feminist health educators were also concerned to present images of women as sexually assertive rather than perpetuating assumptions about female passivity. There

is, however, a very fine line between images that might be seen as 'proactive' and those which appear 'predatory'. I am grateful to my colleagues Kevin Williams and David Miller for providing me with this information from their interviews with those concerned.

References

THE ACT UP/NEW YORK WOMEN AND AIDS BOOK GROUP (1990) *Women, AIDS and Activism,* Boston, South End Press.

BEHARRELL, P. (1993) 'AIDS and the British Press', in ELDRIDGE, J. (Ed.) *Getting the Message,* London, Routledge.

BOFFIN, T. and GUPTA, S. (Eds) (1990) *Ecstatic Antibodies: Resisting the AIDS Mythology,* London, Rivers Oram.

BRANDT, A. (1985) *No Magic Bullet: A Social History of Venereal Disease in the United States since 1880,* Oxford, Oxford University Press.

CLARK, D. (1988) 'AIDS and the Family' *New Society,* 27 May.

JUHASZ, A. (1990) 'The Contained Threat: Women in Mainstream AIDS Documentary', *Journal of Sex Research,* vol. 27, no. 1, pp. 25–46.

KITZINGER, J. (1993) 'Understanding AIDS: Researching Audience Understandings of Acquired Immune Deficiency Syndrome', in ELDRIDGE, J. (Ed.) *Getting the Message,* London, Routledge.

KITZINGER, J. and MILLER, D. (1992) '"African AIDS": The Media and Audience Beliefs', in AGGLETON, P., DAVIES, P. and HART, G. (Eds) *AIDS: Rights, Risk and Reason,* London, Falmer Press.

MCGRATH, R. (1990) 'Dangerous Liaisons: Health, Disease and Representation', in BOFFIN, T. and GUPTA, S. (Eds) *Ecstatic Antibodies: Resisting the AIDS Mythology,* London, Rivers Oram.

MILLER, D. and WILLIAMS K. (1993) 'Negotiating HIV/AIDS Information: Agendas, Media Strategies and the News' in ELDRIDGE, J. (Ed.) *Getting the Message,* London, Routledge.

MORGAN, R. (Ed.) (1970) *Sisterhood is Powerful,* New York, Random House.

THE PLANNING PARTNERSHIP (1988) *HEA/AIDS: A Report on the Qualitative Evaluation of the Health Education Authority AIDS Campaign,* unpublished report.

RHODES, D. and MCNEILL, S. (Eds) (1985) *Women against Violence against Women,* London, Onlywomen Press.

RHODES, T. and SHAUGHNESSY, R. (1990) 'Compulsory Screening: Advertising AIDS in Britain, 1986–89', *Policy and Politics,* vol. 18, no. 1, pp. 55–61.

SMART, C. and SMART, B. (Eds) (1978) *Women, Sexuality and Social Control,* London, Routledge and Kegan Paul.

SMITH, B. (Ed.) (1983) *Home Girls: A Black Feminist Anthology,* New York, Kitchen Table Press.

TREICHLER, P. (in press) 'AIDS Narratives on Television: Whose Story?' in MURPHY, T. and POIRIER, S. (Eds) *Writing AIDS,* New York, Columbia Press.

WELLINGS, K. and ORTON, S. (1988) *Evaluation of the HEA Public Education Campaign, Feb-June, 1988,* unpublished paper.

Section III

Masculinities/Femininities

Chapter 7

Women Have Feelings Too: The Mental Health Needs of Women Living with HIV Infection

Sally Dowling

Introduction

The social construction of HIV infection and AIDS as a predominantly male disease has been well documented elsewhere. This has clear repercussions for women's experience of living with HIV infection, including initial delay in diagnosis, treatment with drugs tested on men only, and a lack of service provision catering for the needs of women. In particular, the mental health needs of women living with HIV infection appear to be poorly understood and not adequately addressed, and it is this issue which is the focus for this chapter. I will first give a brief outline of the main issues, and then go on to critically examine current resources.

The Mental Health Needs of Women Living with HIV Infection

The mental health needs of people living with HIV infection are, to some extent, universal. For example, the shock of being diagnosed HIV-positive, and the need to work through possible feelings of guilt, denial, fear, anxiety and depression are common to both women and men. So too is the stigma attached to HIV and AIDS. However, all aspects of life are gendered. Women may find it easier to express their emotional reactions, and may experience the physical changes of HIV infection as more stigmatizing.

> The effect of having visible lesions in the case of a disease which
> is socially stigmatizing should not be underestimated . . . given

that — far more than men — women are frequently judged in terms of how they look, such changes may be particularly stressful for women. (Richardson, 1989, p. 117).

Alongside these universal issues are concerns which relate specifically to women. These include the invisibility of women living with HIV infection, how HIV/AIDS impacts on lesbian women, the relationship of HIV and AIDS to women's caring, childbearing and childcare roles, and the lack of appropriate service provision for women.

The invisibility of women living with HIV infection has an important effect on women's experiences. Because the reality of heterosexual transmission of HIV infection is not yet widely accepted, women may experience a delay in being offered the test. The shock of discovering HIV-positive status is amplified for many women who have never considered themselves to be at risk, or been informed that heterosexual activity constitutes risk behaviour.

What was weird was the fact that I continued to be examined for six months by three doctors and none of them was able to tell me what was wrong with me (Tema Luft, in Rieder and Ruppelt, 1989, p. 47).

My family doctor laughed when I suggested getting tested for HIV a couple of years ago, and wouldn't test me. He thought that since I was in a monogamous relationship, I was the least at risk. (Penny, in Rieder and Ruppelt, 1989, p. 70).

In November 1991 a woman at an AIDS conference explained how she had visited doctor after doctor for five years, with what she now knows to be symptoms of HIV infection. It was not until she was admitted to hospital, seriously ill with *Pneumocystis carinii* pneumonia (PCP) — an 'AIDS-defining illness' — that she was offered an HIV antibody test and her symptoms were correctly diagnosed (woman at Avon AIDS week conference 'Sharing the Challenge', Bristol, 25 November 1991).

Lesbian women have experienced very different forms of oppression in relation to the issue of HIV. At the beginning of the epidemic, a resurgence of public homophobia was directed at lesbians as well as gay men and they were assumed, particularly by the media, to be similarly 'dangerous'. For example, lesbians have been told of blood transfusion services that do not accept blood they have donated (Richardson, 1989, p. 69). For much of the history of the epidemic, lesbians have been assumed to be at risk. Although it may be true that as a group lesbians are the least 'at risk', some have been infected by a variety of routes, and continue to practise behaviours likely to risk infection of others.

Women with HIV infection are not exempt from the usual gender stereotyping which defines women primarily in relation to their role and their relationship with other people. Women may still be expected to care for others and safeguard their health, even when they themselves are ill. This has been described as 'triple jeopardy' (Panos Institute, 1990). Many women experience their own infection, while worrying about possible infection of their children as well as looking after other infected people.

The majority of women who are infected with HIV, worldwide, are at an age when they are under strong social and cultural pressure to bear children. Indeed, reports suggest that up to 60 per cent of HIV-positive women learn of their own diagnosis only when their children are diagnosed with AIDS. The discovery of HIV-positive status is obviously of key importance to women's decisions concerning whether or not to have children. Some HIV-positive women may decide not to have children. However, most are under strong pressures to see motherhood as part of their role. Grief for their inability to realize their potential may be something that HIV-positive women need particular help in coming to terms with.

> The prospect of not being able to have children was — for me — at least as daunting as the possibility of a premature death. I needed the support of other women who had been through a similar process of saying goodbye to a future with children. (Amanda Heggs, in Panos, 1990, p. iv).

For other women, the choice to have a child may be one of the few positive elements remaining in their lives. One US AIDS researcher has commented on this, saying:

> For many women, childbearing is seen as life-affirming in the face of poverty, drug use, racism, and perhaps the loss of other children to foster care or AIDS. In addition, even a 50 per cent perinatal transmission rate is perceived by some women as an acceptable risk. (Laurie Hauer, quoted in Panos, 1990, p. 47).

In some cultures women who do not bear children have no social role and may be ostracized; in this situation women may feel that they have no choice whether or not to have children. For many women who have little or no say over whether to have sexual intercourse, or whether this is protected or unprotected, real choices and decisions concerning childbearing are also denied.

Women who are already pregnant when they are diagnosed, or who become so afterwards, may find that counselling focuses on the risk to the baby, rather than on the mother's feelings.

> The specialist outlined all the possibilities, which were all horrifying. Not only would my state of health worsen, but, most likely, I would have a sero-positive baby. (Penny, in Rieder and Ruppelt, 1989, p. 72).

The risks of vertical transmission (mother-to-baby) appear to vary worldwide and are continually being reassessed.

An AIDS diagnosis holds many meanings for people, one of which is the association with sexual promiscuity. This has always had particular meaning, historically and culturally, for women, with the double standard of morality being applied. HIV-positive women are stigmatized by this association with promiscuity and are often held responsible for their infection and that of other members of their family, regardless of the actual route of transmission. Women may not only *feel* to blame, they may be told they *are* to blame and have to live, not only with the feelings that this engenders, but with the social ostracism that may follow. A study in Zaire showed, for example, that 'although HIV-positive wives suspected that their husbands had transmitted the virus to them, the wives were held responsible for their illness and sent back to their families while the husbands began living with other women' (Panos, 1990, p. 49).

The early activism of gay men and the construction of AIDS as a male problem has led to the majority of groups, counselling services, and self-help networks being set up around men's needs (although women can be found in all these situations as supporters, counsellors and carers). This can compound the sense of isolation that a woman needing support can feel. An HIV-positive woman living in an area where all the services have developed around men's needs may find herself the only woman in a support group of men. This can make discussion of her needs, particularly those related to sexuality, difficult. For many women the choice is between accepting the situation, or receiving no support.

> In the beginning it was very difficult for me to go there . . . I said, I'm just going to have to take a deep breath and forget I'm the only woman here. (Patty, in Richardson, 1989, p. 119)

The same situation can apply to support groups for people close to an HIV-positive person. Mothers of HIV-positive sons or daughters may not feel comfortable attending support groups where the majority of other members might be partners of people with HIV (in some areas all the other members could be gay men, a situation unlikely to make a middle-aged woman feel at ease). Yet this may be the only means of help or support apparent to a woman in this situation.

A Critical Review of Resources Addressing Mental Health Needs of Women Living with HIV Infection

Despite the fact that there have been women with HIV from very early on in the epidemic, the mental health needs of these women have been virtually ignored. This is true of both standard counselling texts and women's health manuals. For example, one text used in nationwide training courses for counsellors has a small section on 'Counselling the AIDS patient' (seven pages out of 409-page book). This acknowledges that 'AIDS patients' may be women but the issue of women's needs is not addressed (Kennedy and Charles, 1990). Another book, this time aimed at users of counselling services, calls itself 'a complete consumer guide to counselling today' (Quillam and Grove-Stephenson, 1990). In its 'issues guide', under AIDS it does not mention women's needs, although it does include the British Pregnancy Advisory Service in the list of addresses for this section (*ibid.,* p. 182).

One specialist AIDS counselling text (Miller and Bor, 1989) devotes one chapter out of eleven to case discussions, and of these, seven out of twenty-two subjects are women. This is to be welcomed as it does at least make women visible. In most of these case studies women's *specific* needs are not discussed. Instead, women's case studies are used to explore general issues, for example, the testing of blood donors and infection via blood transfusion. The one case study that focuses particularly on women's needs — antibody testing in antenatal clinics (Miller and Bor, 1989, pp. 107–10) — concentrates on the possible risks of infection to others, and neglects the specific emotional or psychological needs of the woman herself. Other specialist AIDS counselling texts do include some material about women, but this is often marginal, being either a very small part of the main text or, as in the example above, not focusing on the *specific* needs of women. Better examples include Anderson and Wilkie (1992), in which there is a chapter about women and AIDS in the section on emotional issues, and the British Association for Counselling/

Department of Health report on HIV counselling (Bond, 1992). This latter text does look, albeit briefly, at women's emotional and psychological needs (although, strangely, it does not index 'women' as a category, even though it does index 'gay men' and 'children'). This report summarizes the specific needs of both infected women and women who are carers, and is almost the only text reviewed that acknowledges that women have specific needs. For example, it states that many women prefer to have a female counsellor, and that some mothers, particularly those with young children, may have difficulty leaving the home for counselling unless some form of childcare facility is provided at the counselling centre. Home visits are a second-best alternative.

Another text, addressing specifically lesbian and gay health care issues, fails to address the issue of women's mental health needs in relation to HIV infection, even though it has a section entitled 'mental health' (Shernoff and Scott, 1988). Even those publications which acknowledge that women's experiences and needs may not be the same as men's neglect women's emotional needs. The Terrence Higgins Trust HIV/AIDS Book (Tavanger, 1992) comments on the exclusion of women from previous accounts about AIDS and discusses issues to do with women and information about physical problems specific to women. There is no information about the emotional needs of women living with HIV infection. Emotional issues are dealt with as if they were gender-neutral. Astonishingly, even the book *Positively Women: Living with AIDS* (O'Sullivan and Thomson, 1992) does not highlight mental health needs as an issue. Feelings and emotions are discussed in individual accounts of living with HIV in the first part of the book. The second part of the book, entitled 'How HIV/AIDS Affects Women's Lives' includes sections on housing, legal needs, pregnancy, sex, and healthy living, but nothing which focuses on psychological needs.

Diane Richardson's *Women and the AIDS Crisis* (1989) is one notable exception. This book recognizes that the problems HIV creates for women are not necessarily the same as for men, and devotes a chapter entitled 'Living with AIDS' to a woman-centred discussion about emotional and psychological needs. This book is a valuable resource, both for women living with HIV, who may find nothing else in print that recognizes their particular needs, and for those who work with women around issues to do with HIV infection.

The Way Forward

It is important to note that there are both individuals and groups who are working with women, raising and addressing mental health issues in an appropriate and sensitive manner. Women-only support groups exist (usually initiated by HIV-positive women), but they tend to be located in large cities and therefore not accessible to all. Where they do exist they provide crucial space in which women can meet their needs for gaining support and information, developing friendships and reducing isolation. Positively Women offers a national telephone helpline and is therefore an important means for enabling women to contact other women with HIV. Health Advisers in Departments of Genito-Urinary Medicine (previously known as sexually transmitted diseases or STD clinics) offer a free confidential service, either by telephone or face to face, to *anyone* concerned about HIV. These clinics are involved in most HIV antibody testing in this country and are often the first point of contact for the newly diagnosed or for those close to someone with HIV. Most Health Advisers are women and, although this does not necessarily place women's mental health on either their personal or professional agenda, it does mean that there are available, in all parts of the UK, female counsellors with knowledge of HIV-related issues.

Conclusion

In summary, therefore, it has been shown that women with HIV infection have many mental health needs. Some of these are specific to women whilst others are experienced in particular ways by women due to their social and cultural position. The social and medical construction of HIV as a health problem for men has direct implications for the health of women living with HIV infection, particularly in their mental health. The awareness in professional and popular literature of their needs is poor, and provision to meet these needs patchy. Women with expertise and knowledge of these issues face an important and urgent task: to raise awareness and focus attention on this (to date) poorly researched area, and to ensure that women everywhere have access to high quality, appropriate, women-focused services. There has recently begun to be an increased professional awareness of the differing *physical* needs of women with HIV; now we need to be aware, and to remember, that women faced with HIV infection have *feelings* too.

Sally Dowling

References

ANDERSON, CHARLES and WILKIE, PATRICIA (1992) *Reflective Helping in HIV and AIDS*, Milton Keynes, Open University Press.
BOND, TIM (1992) *HIV Counselling*, British Association for Counselling/Department of Health report, Rugby, BAC.
FEE, ELIZABETH and FOX, DANIEL M. (Eds) (1988) *AIDS: The Burdens of History*, Berkeley, University of California Press.
HOCKINGS, JACQUELINE (1988) *Walking the Tightrope: Living Positively with AIDS, ARC and HIV*, Loughton, Gale Centre Publications.
KENNEDY, EUGENE and CHARLES, SARA C. (1990) *On Becoming a Counsellor: A Basic Guide for Non-Professional Counsellors*, Dublin, Gill and MacMillan.
MILLER, RIVA and BOR, ROBERT (1989) *AIDS: A Guide to Clinical Counselling*, London, Science Press.
O'SULLIVAN, SUE and THOMSON, KATE (Eds) (1992) *Positively Women: Living with AIDS*, London, Sheba.
PANOS INSTITUTE (1990) *Triple Jeopardy: Women and AIDS*, London, Panos Publications.
QUILLAM, SUSAN and GROVE-STEPHENSON, IAN (1990) *The Counselling Handbook*, Wellingborough, Thorsons.
RICHARDSON, DIANE (1989) *Women and the AIDS Crisis*, 2nd ed., London, Pandora.
RIEDER, INES and RUPPELT, PATRICIA (Eds) (1989) *Matters of Life and Death: Women Speak about AIDS*, London, Virago.
SHERNOFF, MICHAEL and SCOTT, WILLIAM A. (Eds) (1988) *The Sourcebook on Lesbian/Gay Healthcare*, Washington, National Lesbian and Gay Health Foundation Inc.
TAVANYAR, JUDY (1992) *The Terrence Higgins Trust HIV/AIDS Book*, London, Thorsons.
WOMEN IN MIND (1986) *Finding Our Own Solutions*, London, MIND.

Further Reading

AGGLETON, PETER, HART, GRAHAM and DAVIES, PETER (Eds) (1991) *AIDS: Responses, Interventions and Care*, London, Falmer Press.
CLAY, C.J. (1987) *The Social Construction of AIDS*, Sheffield, PAVIC Publications.
CRIMP, DOUGLAS (Ed.) (1988) *AIDS: Cultural Analysis, Cultural Activism*, Cambridge, Mass., MIT Press.
GUNEW, SNEJA (Ed.) (1990) *Feminist Knowledge: (1981) Critique and Construct*, London, Routledge.
HOWELL, ELIZABETH and BAYES, MARJORIE (Eds) (1981) *Women and Mental Health*, New York, Basic Books.
LONDON LESBIAN AND GAY SWITCHBOARD (1992) *Lesbians, HIV and Safer Sex — Low Risk Isn't No Risk*, London, London Lesbian and Gay Switchboard/Health Education Authority.
O'SULLIVAN, SUE (Ed.) (1987) *Women's Health: A Square Rib Reader*, London, Pandora.
PANOS INSTITUTE (1990) *The Third Epidemic: Repercussions of the Fear of AIDS*, London, Panos Publications.
RICHARD, DIANE (1990) *Safer Sex: The Guide for Women Today*, London, Pandora.
SHOWALTER, ELAINE (1987) *The Female Malady: Women, Madness and English Culture, 1830-1980*, London, Virago.

SONTAG, SUSAN (1991) *Illness as Metaphor and AIDS and Its Metaphors,* London, Penguin.

TERRENCE HIGGINS TRUST (1990) *HIV and AIDS: Information for Women,* London, Terrence Higgins Trust (pamphlet).

WILTON, TAMSIN and KANABUS, ANNABEL (Eds) (1990) for AVERT, *Women Talking about AIDS,* Horsham, The AIDS Education and Research Trust.

Chapter 8

Achieving Masculine Sexuality: Young Men's Strategies for Managing Vulnerability

Janet Holland, Caroline Ramazanoglu, Sue Sharpe and Rachel Thomson[1]

Introduction

Sexuality is a central site in men's struggles to become masculine. The dominant cultural ideal of heterosexual masculinity in the UK produces some men as virile, romantic, successful and powerful, but only in relation to others who are not. Western sexuality is characteristically competitive and aggressive, centring on men's desires and men's demonstration of potency. Young men embark on sexual relations with women in social situations in which they are under pressure to become victorious gladiators in the sexual arena, while avoiding the many pitfalls which can reduce them to the ignominy of being a wimp, a failed man, a sexual flop.

We argue that the pressures on young men to achieve particular styles of masculinity require them to exercise power over women, and to define *for* women the nature of sexual encounters. In this chapter, we explore a feminist agenda on women and AIDS by attempting to understand men's struggles to be successfully masculine, and the ways men manage their sexual reputations in their first sexual encounters with women.

Recognition of the power of heterosexual masculinity has, in recent years, been supported by a growing area of studies of masculinity by men (Ramazanoglu, 1992). The feminist perspective which informs much of this research has the effect of problematizing men's heterosexual behaviour. As Arthur Brittan (1989, p. 204) has pointed out, masculinity as a topic did not exist prior to the feminist challenge to male power, since heterosexual men have not conventionally seen themselves as a problem. Vic Seidler has pointed to the invisible man in the discourses of social science (Seidler, 1989, 1991a) and Les Back (1993) muses that he is reminded by the current literature on reflexivity and autobiography of H.G. Wells's character, 'The Invisible Man', who only became visible on his death. It is the feminist challenge to academic discourse that has made the gendered author visible.

Men's studies of men have followed feminism in identifying masculinity as socially constructed, as something which men achieve rather than are born with (Brod, 1987; Kimmel, 1987; Chapman and Rutherford, 1988; Clatterbaugh, 1990; Hearn and Morgan, 1990; Segal, 1990). It is also suggested that, since masculinity can be taken as a social construction, men are not all masculine in the same ways.

David Morgan (1981) proposes that masculinity is not uniform since there are various ways in which men 'do' masculinity, differentiated by sexual identity, class, ethnic and other structural and cultural differences. Carrigan *et al.* (1985) suggest that rather than men conforming to one monolithic version of masculinity, Western cultures produce a dominant or hegemonic masculinity constructed in the image of the white, middle-class, heterosexual male, and differentiated from subordinated masculinities (see also Wight, 1993; forthcoming; Wood, 1987; Nix *et al.*, 1988). An idealized conception of the 'real man' pressures young men to differentiate themselves from gay men, women and failed men.

In the study of young men which we discuss in this chapter, we have found many differences between the young men in the ways they experience their sexuality and their masculinity. Their accounts of their sexuality show them struggling with, attempting to come to terms with, or accepting the constraints, demands and satisfactions of hegemonic, heterosexual masculinity, of becoming 'real' men. The considerable power that is invested in masculinity means that part of being a 'normal' man is the exercise of power over women, whether or not this is recognized, acknowledged or desired by any individual man. From a feminist perspective, we argue that we can identify a tension between the power that men have over women and their own vulnerability to failure as men in the processes of achieving masculine sexuality.

In this chapter we do not oppose the argument that there can be a range of masculinities in a culture, nor that masculinities are culturally constructed and so historically variable. But we are looking for the social factors which explain how men, in spite of their social divisions, weaknesses and vulnerability, continue to exercise such extensive power over women in their sexual relationships. Against the postmodern message that power is everywhere and men do not possess power, we are arguing that men's power is very strongly entrenched in prevailing ideas and institutions, and this has fostered continuity rather than diversity in initial sexual relations. While individual men may be without power, 'man', as a social category to which all individual men have access, to a greater or lesser extent, incorporates structural and cultural power.

In spite of cultural variations in sexuality in recent years, young men's efforts to become 'real men' as they embark on their first sexual encounters with women lead them to exercise considerable power over women, and this power needs to be explained. Here we approach explanation through considering the tensions between young men's vulnerability in forming relationships with women and some key strategies for managing vulnerability through achieving hegemonic masculinity.[2]

The Studies of Young People

Our argument is based on two studies of young people: the Women, Risk and AIDS Project (WRAP) and Men, Risk and AIDS project (MRAP).[3] These studies have generated a large body of qualitative data on the sexual knowledge and practice of young men and women between 1988 and 1992. The first study was of the accounts of their negotiation of sexual encounters given by young women aged 16–21 in London and Manchester. The Men, Risk and AIDS Project (MRAP) was a comparative study of forty-six young men in London between 1991 and 1992.[4]

We aimed in these two studies to build up a detailed picture of the sexual practices, beliefs and understanding of young people; to document and interpret their understanding of HIV and sexually transmitted diseases, their conceptions of risk and danger in sexual activity, their approaches to relationships and responsibility within them, and their ability to communicate effectively their ideas on safety within sexual relationships. It is also our intention to contribute to the development of the theory of the social construction of sexuality, by identifying some of the complexity of the processes and mechanisms through which young people construct, experience and define their sexuality and sexual practices.

The main method of data collection was an in-depth interview conducted in a naturalistic style with the researcher prepared to pursue any issues of particular relevance to the young people themselves. Further qualitative material was provided by detailed field notes of the interviews, covering the context and nature of the interaction and a detailed description of the young person. The sensitivity of the topic area and the difficulties which young people have in finding a language to express their experience of sexual activity renders some of the information which became available to us implicit in the verbal exchange. We attempted to make explicit the implicit in the field notes.[5]

The interview samples were based on the variables of age, ethnicity, socio-economic class, education, and sexual activity. The samples generated in this way for the WRAP study were in fact comparable in relevant sexual activity (levels of sexual activity, age of first sex) to random samples of young people generated in other studies (for example those of Ford and Morgan, 1989; Bowie and Ford, 1989; and Ford, 1991).[6]

In this chapter, we draw on data from the Men, Risk and AIDS Project, but the analysis and interpretation of the data on young women feeds into and illuminates the work that we have done on young men.[7] Where we have quoted from interview transcripts, the young men are identified by a number. This refers the reader to a brief note on the young man in question, contained in the Appendix to this chapter.

Power and Vulnerability

We have interpreted the young men's accounts of their sexuality to argue that there are three main ways in which heterosexual men can be vulnerable in sexual encounters:

(1) First, they may simply fail to measure up to the culturally defined requirements of hegemonic masculinity.

(2) Second, young men are vulnerable, as Seidler (1989) has argued, because negotiating sexual encounters can engage their emotions, connect them to their need for affection, and render visible their dependence on women. Successful masculinity puts them under pressure to conceal the extent of their vulnerability through caring, dependency, loving and any other characteristic of nurturing or effeminacy.

A man laid low by love can be dependent, hurt, dismissed, rejected; he is a man at risk as a man. Much of the new 'men's studies' has emphasized what we term 'men's pain', and the emotional constriction of hegemonic masculinity, which leaves men injured by the demands of masculinity.

(3) Third, men are vulnerable when they enter into sexual relationships with women, because women do not necessarily conform to cultural ideas of subordinated femininity. As

Wendy Hollway has put it (1981, p. 39), 'men measure their masculinity against women's sexuality'. Where women develop their own desires, or resist subordination, their sexuality, the material reality of their bodies and desires, constitute a potential threat to conventional masculinity.

Faced with these threats, there are strategies available to young men to divert or manage their vulnerability. We argue that, despite the reality of 'men's pain', these strategies have the effect of reinforcing and reproducing male power. We focus on four key strategies:

(1) adopting the protective coloration of the peer group;

(2) objectifying and dismissing women in general, and in particular the woman who is the means by which first penetrative sexual experience is acquired (Litewka, 1977);

(3) seeking out a knowing older women from whom to acquire appropriate knowledge;

(4) wielding the weapon of attributing a negative sexual reputation to a woman.

Before looking at these strategies we comment briefly on the ways young men talked about learning about sex as these were rather different from those reported by young women.

Learning about Sex — The Knowing Man

The WRAP team have argued that the cultural context within which young women acquire their knowledge of sex provides no positive model of female sexuality (Thomson and Scott, 1991). The messages they receive are couched in a 'protective discourse' which emphasizes negative outcomes of sexual activity including the dangers of unwanted pregnancy. Available images cast women as passive, victims of male sexuality, and are geared entirely to their reproductive function.

Our data support the view that young men receive less formal sex education than young women (Allen, 1987; Currie, 1990). Although both tend to consider their sex education inadequate and too late, more men do so than women. In fact many of the young men found it difficult to pin down exactly where they had learned about sex.

I think I've always known what would go on in sex. Somebody didn't tell me one day and it was a revelation. I think I've always known from a very early age.

There was a general perception that they 'just knew' about sex, which could be coupled with an acknowledgment of gaps in that knowledge, and of sources of information they had drawn on (Holland, 1993). Their knowledge forms part of a general cultural context in which it is the male construction and definition of heterosexual sex — vaginal penetration with the man as the prime mover and actor — which is the norm.

Both young men and women accepted the prevailing heterosexual definition of sex as male penetration of the vagina, and each assume that this is what men want. The young men in the sample expected, and felt that they were expected, to both want to have sex and to enjoy it. Unlike women, they were offered a positive and active conception of male sexual identity.

Three crucial interrelated differences in the overall context in which women and men learn about sex and their own sexuality help to construct the differences we observe in male and female sexuality, and contribute to unequal gendered power relations in sexual relations:

(1) the male is regarded as the knowing sexual agent and actor; the woman as unknowing and acted upon;

(2) 'normal' heterosexual sex is defined by an act which is seen as meeting male need and desire, and providing pleasure and satisfaction for the male; autonomous female pleasure and desire are largely absent from dominant heterosexual discourses, and women are constructed as gaining satisfaction from meeting men's needs; sex is seen as something men do to women;

(3) men have access to a positive image of active, male sexuality, while women learn about sex through a 'protective discourse' which emphasizes reproductive capacity and the dangers of sexual activity — essentially a negative, passive image of female sexuality.

This image of the knowing man, and the positive conception of an active pleasure-seeking male sexuality, put particular pressures on young men to become 'real men' in their sexual relationships with women.

Strategies for Managing Vulnerability

(1) The Pleasures and Perils of the Peer Group

Faced with social pressures to become sexually active, young men can seek support from their peers through the vicissitudes of the road to masculinity, but this process is complex, and fraught with tensions and contradiction. Young men are potentially vulnerable as sexual and social failures. When young men talk among themselves about their sexual exploits and experiences, they are struggling to establish themselves as acceptably masculine, within a competitive framework. Accounts of peer group talk do seem to support a version of hegemonic masculinity which is clearly differentiated from effeminacy, sensitivity and homosexuality. We have identified, in these reports of talk, what we call performance stories.

Performance Stories
Although there is some awareness among young men of the need to keep within certain parameters of credibility when they talk about sex, the content of male talk about their sexual activities need bear little relation to their experience. There is a common acceptable of such stories as including exaggeration and even lying, which is not necessarily publicly challenged, although it can contribute to a reputation as a wimp or, as in this case, an idiot:

> A: When you've got a gathering in a mate's house, and then it comes round to me — 'What did you do?' and I say 'I had sex, so what'. They say, 'have you done this?', and 'do you fancy this girl?', you know what I mean. They do my head in, I don't really mix with them now.
> Q: And do people tell the truth . . .
> A: Most of them lie, most of them anyway.
> Q: What, to give a good impression!
> A: I think they do. 'Ah, I did it ten times last week' — everyone knows he's lying but he still says it, some people think he's a bloody idiot. (YM 6)

Behind the boasting and exaggeration lies the dominant conception of heterosexual masculinity to which the young men aspire or from which they fear they may fall short. Acceptance and collusion can play a part in assessing the competition, and placing oneself in the performance.

Q: And did you discuss that sort of thing a lot?

A: Well, it all depends whether anybody had a girlfriend. If you had a girlfriend it was talked about, if you didn't you basically steered clear of the problem. I suppose it killed a lunchtime just talking about it. You often got the bloke who was making it up as he went along because he would contradict himself halfway through, but you still listened because he might know something that you don't know, and you are eager to find out what he does know.

Q: Did you point out that he had made a contradiction and things like that?

A: Basically we just let him finish and then we would take it with a pinch of salt whatever he said, some of it may be true, it may all be lies, but we just leave him, if that's what he wants to think there is no point in us breaking up his dreams or whatever. He went to the bother of telling us, we might as well leave him, if that's what he thought.

Q: Have you ever done that yourself?

A: I have got to admit I told one or two porkers a couple of times. Basically you are always in the playground and everybody's there and they have all got a story, and you are standing there and you have got no story, so when it actually comes round to you, you decide to make up a little bit, or if you have been out with a girl in the past, you just change her name and change a couple of things about her so they think it's somebody else, which works sometimes, but other times I had the feeling they knew . . . (YM 7)

But the performance stories of others can conflict with a young man's own experience:

A: . . . now I know he lied because he said 'yes, yes, it was great', that was like the first time he lost his virginity and I'm sure he was lying because he was just saying how wonderful it was and I don't think it is that wonderful. I think he was just saying that because everyone presumes it is, everyone just presumes it's just the best thing, it's not really. (YM 2)

The reverse can also happen, when an actual sexual experience or encounter can be seen by the young man as unbelievable to his friends, so that he would hesitate to tell them for fear of being disbelieved, and perhaps ridiculed. (We return to this point below).

Our point is that performance stories function to establish a young man's position in the competition to be a 'real man', and to create and sustain a particular sexual image. Male fantasy and bravado expressed in performance stories help to define and reproduce the male model of sexuality to which young men are expected to aspire. At the same time, these stories can challenge, as well as reinforce, the acquisition of masculinity.

Young men generally characterized stories as entailing some element of boasting, exaggeration or lies. In our interpretation, it was important for them to be able to treat stories in this way, as a means of keeping sexual competition at a manageable level. If the stories were taken to be true, the performer could emerge as sexual superman and so victorious in the peer group competition. Performance stories undermine men with no sexual experience or lesser exploits to report, while maintaining collective masculinity. Ridicule from peers serves as an instrument of control to ensure that the ideal of male heterosexuality is pursued.

Competition, Pressure and Ridicule

When young men talk amongst themselves about their sexual exploits and experiences, they are not primarily seeking to gain knowledge about sex and sexuality, but attempting to create and reproduce a certain image of themselves. In this competition to demonstrate acceptable masculinity, to prove themselves as men, the image they must present is of a macho, knowing, and experienced male.

> Q: Tell me more about these sort of roles that are forced onto men. What those may be in terms of having sex?
> A: Well they tend to be rather crude. I was in a rugby club when I was twelve or thirteen and the older rugby club members would go on about sex. From the way they were talking you would get the impression that as long as you were sticking your dick up somebody then you should be happy and that was all there was to it. And you really didn't have to feel anything for the person, in fact you shouldn't really feel anything for the person at all. (YM 8)

This is a succinct definition of what we term 'the male model of sexuality'. This is a model which identifies male power as sexual conquest over women and separation from emotional involvement with them (a model which can also be adopted by women: see Holland *et al.*, 1992a).

This male model operates as a defence against the vulnerability of emotional involvement with a partner, but also creates vulnerability in the extent to which young men fall short of this ideal of male heterosexuality.[8]

A: I know. It's just the . . . it's just the think like . . . it's like I think of it as all men are gladiators, right, and the more competitions they win with women, the more stronger they feel. (YM 9).

Competition in one form or another plays an integral role in the acquisition of masculinity, and several of these young men referred to a competition to lose their virginity:

A: there was a group of four of us, really, really close friends and I was like the first person to lose my virginity out of them. I think they were shocked because I had lost my virginity and they hadn't, like I think everyone had the idea that they would lose theirs first and it was like they . . . I don't know, I think that was partly why I wanted to do it as well, like it was a competition. (YM 2)

The competitive pressure continues as the sexual career progresses:

A: it's a big image problem everyone's got with sex. It's got to be high, you have got to have sex all the time, sleep with loads of different girls, it's like that.
Q: Yes, and do you think guys still feel that way?
A: I think it is a bit of a competition all the time. (YM 2)

For young men, success in this competition is sexual conquest, and the audience for this victory is the male peer group rather than the sexual partner:

Q: Do you think that sex means something different for the boys and for the girls?
A: Yes, definitely, men just see it as something that has got to be done, that's what I think, so your friends don't tease you. Women see it as something that really means something to them. We are using them to get something, I don't know, it's all ego when it comes down to it for the men . . . it's like an achievement. (YM 5)

The male peer group can exert pressure and employ ridicule, 'taking the mickey', to keep young men on the straight and narrow path towards heterosexual masculinity. A positive image is created by professing to have had sex with a girl, and even better, by having a 'good fuck' with a desirable girl.

In these groups, young men are subjected to teasing, having the mickey taken, and forms of collective pressure to express and define themselves in a particular way in order to prove their manhood. Aggression too can be seen in the negative labelling of those who fall short, or whose sexual claims are not believed — 'wimps', 'wallies' and 'wankers'. What the group does seem to support is a particular concept of hegemonic heterosexual masculinity, and separation from effeminacy, or homosexuality.

The threat of sexual failure can turn a potential gladiator into a wimp. The following young man discusses in some detail the tensions and pain in having gained a reputation as a wimp, and the complex way in which the apparently joking attribution can act as a spur to performance:

Q: Why do boys want so much sex?

A: Maybe like because they have got friends that act this way like, they just want one thing and they like the idea really and they try to do it themselves and stuff like that, I mean they just copy each other really.

Q: So when you said earlier something about boys having a reputation, is that what you mean?

A: Yes.

Q: What do their mates think of them?

A: Like supposing if they go to a party and meet a girl and nothing happens, then the guy's a wimp and stuff like that.

Q: Do you think their mates actually mean that or they just do it?

A: They do it to wind them up like.

Q: But it still –

A: Yes, it still, like, hurts, it gets on your inside and like the person knows next time he has got to do it.

Q: It's funny, if when they call somebody a wimp they don't really mean it.

A: It's just really to give them a boost like. But the person who has been called that doesn't know what, sort of thing, but it just builds him up for the next time, he knows what to do. (YM 3)

This young man had indeed suffered from teasing from his friends, and when he eventually lost his virginity, it was more for their benefit than this own:

A: At the time I was at school — they used to say the only time you would get off with a girl is when she is deaf, blind and stuff like that and that's where the feeling came from — 'if only my friends could see me now'.

Q: So you felt you had to prove yourself?

A: Yes.

Q: Why was that? Did you actually believe that they thought you were inadequate in some way?

A: Yes. Most of them take the mickey out of you and stuff like that and so you are more determined and so you feel you have to do it to prove yourself to them.

Q: But isn't it only a joke when they take the mickey out of you?

A: Most of the time it is, but it still hurts though, and it's just as bad as if they were serious.

Q: It's a funny thing to do to your friends isn't it?

A: Well it is and it isn't. Like most of them said it when I used to be at school like, one told me it's for your own good that people take the mickey out of you, the boy that told me was in the sixth form so he was much older, and he told me that, it's only for your own good and stuff like that. It makes you more determined to go out there and do it.

Young men facing failure in the eyes of their peers can redeem themselves by losing their virginity, or gaining sexual access to any girl who can be passed off as desirable. The strategies adopted in defence of their sexual reputation suggest that a harsh dichotomy is produced between the possibilities of becoming a wimp or a gladiator.

(2) A Hit and Run Affair: The 'Bastard' Syndrome

One strategy used by the young men for dealing with the tensions and problems associated with losing virginity was to adopt the 'male model' of heterosexuality, in which, as we heard earlier, the woman is an object of male power and conquest, with no concern for her as a person, and the main objective is penetrative sex.[9] This can be seen as a strategy for exercising power and protecting oneself from vulnerability, yet it comes at the cost of a limited conception of sexuality. A number of young men in the study employed this approach for their first experience of sex. In the following case it involves seeing loss of virginity as a one-off experience to be accomplished as soon and as speedily as possible, a rite of passage with little concern for the woman. There were quite a number of young men in the sample for whom this self-protective technique appeared to work, and they saw behaving in this way as an important part of masculine sexuality. In their view, who you had intercourse with was less important for men than for women:

> A: I think from a bloke's point of view they are not so bothered like who they lose their virginity to, or who they sleep with, and I think to a girl, or woman it means a lot more. (YM 2)

And another (asked about whether he felt different on losing his virginity):

> A: I mean I think it is — I know it's a cliché but — I think it's a much bigger event in women's lives. (YM 2)

This belief helped to boost their masculinity by distancing them from any feelings for the woman and concern for her feelings, in that if a woman was prepared to have sex after limited acquaintance, she fell short of the standard of ideal feminine sexuality.

> Q: Was it her first time?
> A: She said it was but I — I don't know whether it was or not. 'Cos like it was too quick like for her like, for a girl to say it was, like in a couple of hours. It would have been more if like if she was a virgin, so I reckon she wasn't. (YM 12)

A sense of emotional distance came through very directly in some of the interviews:

> A: It didn't really bother me at all. It's not as though you lose anything really is it? It's just something in your mind, suddenly you know that you're not a virgin any more. (YM 13)

Another young man had picked up some girls at a club with his friend and it happened in the back of his friend's father's car:

A: We went to a club to meet some girls and met them and that was that really. There's not a lot I can say about that. It was fun, but it wasn't anything more serious, I've seen her, but I have never spoken to her since . . . I saw her again but I never spoke to her again. I've no hang-ups about that. (YM 11).

The 'hit and run' approach, reducing women to a subordinated 'other', is consistent with the pressures to lose virginity and compete in performance stories. It has more complicated ramifications when adopted as a way of life. The young man quoted above (YM 11) continued his sex life in a similar style, having one-night stands or short relationships, enjoying the chase more than anything else. He would then tire of the girl and move on. In his own report he has acquired the reputation of being uncaring, arrogant and hard, even amongst his friends.

The existence of the gladiatorial 'bastard' can make life even more difficult for the self-confessed 'wimp'. One young man described the difficulties of being 'nice'; he felt that women preferred 'bastard guys' since at least they asked women out. For 'bastard guys' rejection was not much of a problem; if one woman refused you just moved on and put your request to the next one. Nice guys found it difficult to approach women at all because more of their 'selves' were involved, and rejection was therefore harder to bear:

A: most women seem to find sort of bastard guys attractive you know, the ones the ones that sleep around and — simply because they're the only ones that ever ask people out, you know, try and chat people up.
Q: What, so you think the nicer guys lose out?
A: Yeah I think they do. Simply because, I don't know, say, if you just go for a basic asking out you know, on a date, people who are more say, either romantic, or less interested in sex and more interested in a relationship have a lot at stake when they ask someone. You know, they've got all their emotional attributes at stake. You know, when they say — 'look do you wanna go out Friday night?' they've got, you know 'do you want to spend time with me? Do you like me as a person? Do you –?' you know, blah, blah, blah. Obviously 'Do you find me attractive?', but 'Do you like me?' Whereas the sort of bastard guys who are quite happy to

sleep with anyone you know, if they say 'Do you wanna go out tonight?' bascially meaning you know, 'Do you wanna go out for a drink -- then we'll go back to my house, we'll have sex, we'll go away and we'll never talk to each other again'. You know, they've got nothing to lose if someone says no, you know — 'Fine. How about you?' — they can just keep going on. (YM 4)

Sexual success on the terms of the bastard syndrome does not necessarily render men invulnerable. In some cases, when 'the bastard syndrome' characterized a young man's sexual strategy, and women were successfully objectified, vulnerability could be revealed as providing the motor for such behaviour. One young man had been hurt by a girl for whom he did not particularly care, but who finished with him. After this experience he made sure that he was the one who decided to end relationships to protect himself from possible pain:

A: If a girl broke off a relationship with me then I would tend to be a little bit hurt, where I thought it was better if I broke it off with her, it wouldn't hurt so much. If I found another girlfriend pretty soon it would help me forget about it and it didn't hurt me as much. (YM 10)

He preferred to have short, sexual relationships:

A: I was lucky because as I left one, it was only a matter of days or a week and I was into another relationship because I used to go out quite a lot then, clubs and that.

He did not care for any of these girlfriends, it was just something to do, slipping easily from one relationship to the next. He never really knew, or bothered to find out, what the girls involved thought or felt, but he did manage to polish his technique by enquiring what they liked.

A: I tend to ask some girlfriends what they prefer sort of thing, and try and do that to them.
Q: And what do you find they do prefer?
A: A bit more caring and a bit more slowly, not just get undressed and do it and just sit there. They tend to like it a bit more caring and lovingly, even though I didn't love them. I did try to keep them happy.

But now he has been laid low, or perhaps raised up, by love. He is in love with his current girlfriend:

> A: I'm more understanding towards women now, I'm less sexist as well for some reason, I don't know why . . . It has changed me a lot, yes I've grown up another couple of years in the space of about five months. It's really helped me a lot.

Sex used just to be vaginal intercourse but now:

> A: When you are in a long-term relationship you care about someone, you do want to make love, it feels different. It feels totally different . . . But now my girlfriend, because I love her and that, we can actually make love without actually having intercourse, just being nice to one another and that and just haven't got intercourse, but it feels we are making love. But with other girlfriends sex had to be intercourse, so it was sex.

This young man's experience illustrates the limits of the bastard syndrome. The pursuit of this model causes men to miss out on all areas of sexuality and desire which are more than intercourse, while ostensibly protecting them from vulnerability and pain. The syndrome demonstrates a direct exercise of male power, in which at the same time (as contributors to Seidler (1991b) have argued) men suffer from the limits of masculinity.

(3) The Knowing Woman: Seduction and the Older Woman

We have seen that the sexually knowing man is the norm. The knowing woman can represent both threat and promise for young men on the route to heterosexual masculinity, and she appears in two of the strategies which can be used to divert vulnerability.

The third strategy available to young men for ridding themselves of the burden of virginity (recognizing their own vulnerability in the process) is to surrender to the superior knowledge and desire of the older woman. Here too the physical and emotional risks of sex, or even a relationship, with another virgin are being avoided. This surrender to seduction is simultaneously a conquest, and a consummation devoutly to be wished,[10] so much so that a number of the young men who had this experience either did not tell their mates because they assumed their stories would not be believed, or told them, unbothered by disbelief, because they were secure in their own knowledge and satisfaction. Holidays, one-off sexual encounters and short relationships character-ized this type of sexual initiation.

One young man (aged 15) had been in a pub and was invited back to a woman's home to help her with a repair problem.

> A: I went into the bedroom and she was naked on the bed. I went 'Um, my god!', because I kind of like froze, there was this woman, a good seventeen years my senior just sprawled out on the bed with nothing on. I had often seen the odd porno mag like and seen it, but when you actually see it really, you kind of go 'oh!' for the first time. (YM 7)

He was not sure of her motivation,

> A: but basically she just instructed me on what to do, and I had to do things . . . she just talked me through it. It was really strange . . .
> A: I went round for the next four days with a great big smile on my face. . . .
> A: I will remember that as long as I live.

He was afraid his friends would not believe him:

> A: I told a couple of my mates at school after a little while, I thought sod it, I will, they can take the mick they don't have to believe me. I know within myself that I have actually done it, so if they don't believe me, they don't have to.

A night in a tent at the age of 14 with an older, experienced woman evoked similar fears of peer group ridicule for another young man:

> A: I did talk to a few close friends about it, but the first time I didn't want to tell too many people because to say you lost your virginity to a girl on holiday in a tent it's just so unbelievable, like it's not worth it — everyone is going to turn round and go 'oh yes?', so I kept that pretty quiet at the time, just like there was no point in saying, it sounds such a dodgy story. (YM 2)

One young man was desperate to lose his virginity:

> A: I just wanted to get older so that I could have sex. Childhood wasn't very interesting actually. (YM 1)

At 14 he had a two-week holiday sexual relationship with a 19-year-old:

> A: I mean I couldn't have handled losing my virginity to another virgin because you wouldn't have a clue about what was going on, you know. So at least I've learned a few things, you know.

Acknowledging superior knowledge in women was not always experienced unproblematically, and this young man was loath to abandon the idea of the sexually knowing male:

> Q: So did she kind of teach you almost, show you what –
> A: No, she didn't. I mean, you know it just, to a certain extent you know what to do by the time it comes. But obviously she did a bit of guiding, you know, but er, yeah, I wasn't totally ineffectual anyway.

The knowing older woman can be acceptable and sought after by young men, even if experiencing vulnerability may prove problematic.[11] Daniel Wight (personal communication) has questioned whether young men can be taken to be exercising power in relationships with older women. We do not mean to argue here that the seduction of a young man by an older woman necessarily enables a direct exercise of male power over this woman. If power relations are socially constructed, male power is never assured. In the WRAP study of young women some young women, who had had negative sexual experiences with men, employed the strategy of only having relationships with younger men. This, they felt, gave them more power to control both the sex and the relationship (Holland *et al.*, 1991). Young men can use sexual initiation by older women to manage their own vulnerability in their more general struggle to become successfully masculine.

The knowing female friend, with whom they can discuss the intricacies of relationships and seek advice and comfort, also figures widely in the experience of the young men in the sample. In this case she need not necessarily be sexually experienced herself, but can provide information about the physical aspects of women's bodies (including periods, a subject on which many of the young men required schooling), and emotional aspects of relationships, from the woman's perspective. Mothers and older sisters could sometimes fulfil this function. The knowing younger woman is an altogether different matter.

(4) 'Slag' - Sexual Reputation and the Double Standard

Having sexual experience or expressing active sexual desires puts a young woman in danger of acquiring a 'slack' reputation as a slag. The fear of such a reputation can exercise strong control over a young woman's sexual experience and identity (Lees, 1993; Thomson and Scott, 1991; Holland *et al.*, 1991). Young women must tread the treacherous line between losing their reputation through engaging in sexual activity, or losing a desired social status conferred by 'having a boyfriend', where sex is part of the relationship. When men are known for their sexual prowess it is seen as a gain in reputation; if women are known for their sexual activity, it is seen as a loss in reputation. As one of the young women in the WRAP study put it:

> with girls you're brought up to be ladylike, 'cos if you start being rampant you're called a slag or a slut or whatever, but with boys they can get away with anything, like they won't really get called no major names, they just get called Casanova and things like that, but that's not really gonna hurt them, like if a girl gets called a slag.

For young men, the power of being able to attribute a negative reputation to the sexually knowing woman can counterbalance the vulnerability of exposing themselves to her capacity for comparison. This strategy is related to the male model of masculinity and objectification of women, and we have given examples of how the attribution of experience to young women can enable this objectifying approach in the 'bastard syndrome' discussed earlier. Young men who believe that a man has to prove himself as a 'gladiator' are made vulnerable by the possibility of feedback about their performance.

> A: I have never asked someone afterwards, 'was it good for you?' because if they said, 'well, actually . . .' I'd die.

This conception of the need for men to be both dominant and sexually successful encourages young men to objectify and denigrate women since women can threaten their masculinity. Men have to prove their prowess to women as well as report it back to men.

Q: Do you think that men are more nervous of women, or women more nervous of men?

A: I think men are more nervous than women because they are the ones that have got something to prove like, sort of thing, so I think like men have got to be a bit more nervous than women in a way.

Q: So in reality it is women who are in the more dominant position?

A: Yes, because they have got to like — they sort of like assess the performance sort of thing, if you get what I mean, afterwards they say I was lousy and something like that. The men have to prove to them that they are capable of doing it with them . . .

Q: Is there a sort of feeling do you think amongst men to think they have to be good at sex?

A: I think so yes, especially if you have seen the girl about and stuff like that, and like you know she is going to open her mouth to everyone else if you are not good, so yes, you have to perform quite well if you know the girl like, and you have seen her about.

Q: Does that make you quite nervous thinking you have to perform quite well?

A: Sometimes it does (YM 3)

The pressure to identify some women as slags is also related to the presence of peer pressure. The following young man recognizes a double standard:

Q: Since women are changing do you think it's okay for the woman to make the first approach?

A: I think it would help a lot of men out if they did.

Q: You don't think they are though?

A: Some are. I think it helps a great deal if they do, I think it's just something born out of like what people think should happen. Women probably feel that they shouldn't really make the first move because the men are going to think something of them that they shouldn't do.

Q: You think they might think badly of them?

A: Yes I think that happens quite a bit, which is a shame really, because it's like the old thing that if the man makes the first move he's just looked at in a different light to what if the woman did the same thing. (YM 14)

This young man is quite happy for his own girlfriend to make the first moves, but it appears to be her age which makes it acceptable:

A: That's just due to an age gap, she's like twenty-five so it doesn't bother me. It's actually nice for me for all the right reasons.

Perhaps he would not be quite so happy if his girlfriend was the same age.[12] Other young men who consider that it is hard for men to make the first move, and that it would be helpful if girls did so, express more contradictory views:

A: Like girls always expect blokes to make the first move, I think that's a pretty common thought and if they want to be equal then they should make the first move as well, but they never do and that's fairly frustrating from a bloke's point of view.

Q: Then how might you feel about a girl if a girl came on to you?

A: I always sit there and I always consider it to myself . . . I would say yes, that would be all right . . . (he is expressing this view rather doubtfully)

Q: It might be related to this slag thing, because they feel that if they make the first move the guy's going to think they want sex, they must be a slag, do you think that's the way it works out?

A: Yes, it would, because if the girl made a big move on me I would just take it as a big come-on, I would presume they wanted sex. (YM 2)

A distinction between sex and love was identified by the young women in the WRAP study, but on the whole the young women worked hard at integrating the two. Maintaining a distinction between 'fucking' and 'making love', however, was central to much of the young men's discussion of sexuality. For many of the young men there clearly were girls with whom you had sex — as opposed to a relationship — and putting pressure on them to have sex was a legitimate part of the process.

A young woman describes this from her perspective:

> If a girl sleeps with him and if she consents quickly to the boy
> saying, 'Yeah, I'll have sex with you', then he'll think she's slack
> whereas if a girl says, 'No', sometimes he'll say to her 'Oh, you're
> frigid', but in his mind he'll be thinking, 'She's a bit sensible. She
> knows what she's thinking'. But he'll try and make her feel bad.
> Whereas a girl, if she goes to bed with him, he'll say, 'Oh yeah,
> you're lovely', then the next day he'll be calling her a slag behind
> her back.

The ability to label a woman a slag (which is also widely used by
young women against each other, to preserve their own reputations)
gives young men considerable power to manage their vulnerability and
protect themselves from appraisal by knowing younger women. But the
related need to be 'good at sex' distances young men from perceiving
masculinity in terms of negotiated, balanced and caring relationships. It
feeds into a competitive and limited conception of male sexuality in
which men can become sexually 'successful', while cutting themselves off
from emotional dependence. The young gladiator then wields a two-
edged sword — proving his manhood to himself and his peers, while
cutting the ground of positive relationships from beneath himself.

Conclusion: Vulnerability and Power

Young men were generally aware that in entering into the negotiation of
sexual encounters they were laying themselves open to the possibility of
failure. We consider that their strategies for dealing with their potential
vulnerability tended to reproduce and reinforce the exercise of male
power over women. The exercise of male power can act directly against
women's sexual safety. It is not that men necessarily insist on unsafe
sexual practice, but the 'logic' of male-defined sex makes the negotiation
of sexual safety problematic.

Young men's struggles to be successfully masculine, to emerge as
young gladiators rather than as wimps, involve them in defining their
sexuality in terms of male needs, male desires and male satisfactions,
rather than in terms that might acknowledge and engage with female
sexuality, and their own emotions and dependence. The way in which
this competition for masculinity is played out protects men from
acknowledging a subtext of men's fears of an independent female
sexuality.

Fear is not generally expressed directly in the transcripts, but is implied obliquely in the defensive strategies with which young men protect their masculinity from the power of women's desires, and from dependence on women. Where young men resist the pressures of masculinity by developing emotional and caring relationships with women which put their masculinity at risk, they are still aware of, and measured against, the image of young gladiators.

We would not rule out the possibility of the 'new man' or what we would call the 'willing wimp' being aware of, and being able to deconstruct, power relationships, but the willing wimp still operates sexually in social contexts that empower the male in relation to the female. Whether or not individual young men achieve or resist hegemonic masculinity, or develop sub-cultural styles of masculinity, the social processes which constitute 'becoming a man' shore up the enormous strength of men's sexual domination of women, and do this across men's social differences. In these processes men can certainly suffer pain, humiliation, loss, ridicule and rejection, yet both wimps and gladiators exist in a framework of social relations that demand the exercise of male power over women.

We need to note that young women very generally also define sexuality in terms of male privilege. In producing themselves as feminine, and accepting men's power to define what sort of sexual encounter they are entering into, young women can *enable* even wimpish men to exercise power over them (Holland *et al.*, 1992a, 1992b). The 'embedding of safer sex practice within relationship structures and understandings' which has been observed among middle-class, white, gay men (Davies *et al.*, 1993, p. 175) requires levels of communication and negotiation which are very difficult for young people to achieve within the current framework of hegemonic heterosexual masculinity, and its subordinated femininity.

Cultural resistance is possible, but young men embarking on their first sexual encounters are generally in a contradictory situation in which they suffer from being socially pressured into a narrow and constraining conception of masculine sexuality, but they also benefit from social arrangements which systematically privilege male sexuality, desire and prowess.

Appendix

YM1 Aged 21.   Lives with friends in student house. Studying for a degree at university.

YM2 Aged 16.   Lives at home with parents, brother and sister.

YM3 Aged 16.   Lives at home with parents and brothers. Attending training agency; looking for youth training course.

YM4 Aged 18.   Lives at home with parents and brother. About to start a degree at university after a year off.

YM5 Aged 17.   Lives at home with mother, three brothers and a sister. At sixth-form college studying for 'A' Levels.

YM6 Aged 16.   Lives at home with father and stepmother. Attending training agency. Wants to be a motor mechanic.

YM7 Aged 20.   Lives at home with parents and brother. Works as an engineer.

YM8 Aged 21.   Lives on his own. Studying for a degree at university.

YM9 Aged 18.   Lives at home with mother, brother and sister. Works at night replacing stock in a store.

YM10 Aged 17.   Lives at home with parents. Attending training agency; wants to be a motor mechanic.

YM11 Aged 17.   Lives at home with mother, stepfather, stepbrother and sister. At school studying for 'A' Levels.

YM12 Aged 18.   Lives at home with parents and two sisters. At school studying for GCSE and 'A' Levels.

YM13 Aged 19.   Lives at home with parents. Works as an engineer. Studying for City and Guilds on day release.

YM14 Aged 19.   Lives at home with parents. Just left school after taking 'A' levels; looking for advertising job.

Notes

1   We are grateful for the contribution of Tim Rhodes to the work on which this paper is based.
2   The relationship between the exercise and experience of power in a heterosexual sexual encounter and the broad societal institutionalization of male power remains to be explained. In early sexual relations, where there is often little communication and much ambiguity, male power may not be exercised directly, but it still structures the sexual encounter (see Kent *et al.*, 1990).
3   The Women, Risk and AIDS Project study of young women was staffed by the authors and Sue Scott, now at the University of Stirling, and was financed by a two-year grant from the ESRC. Additional funding was contributed by the Department of Health and Goldsmiths' College Research Fund. Valuable assistance has been given by Jane Preston, Polly Radcliffe and Janet Ransom.

   The Leverhulme Trust gave a one-year grant for the study of young men, and Tim Rhodes, now at the Centre for Research on Drugs and Health Behaviour, was a team member on this second project. The study included interviews with advisors on sexuality to young people.
4   Access to the young people was gained through a range of settings, including work, training, educational, leisure and health organizations. The young people were invited to complete a questionnaire, and to provide a name and contact address if they wished to take part in an interview study. The young men were asked if they would prefer a male or female interviewer, or had no preference.
5   The problems of uncertainty in interpreting interview data are discussed in Holland and Ramazanoglu (forthcoming).
6   The interviews were transcribed into a form appropriate for the use of the Ethnograph, a computer program developed to ease the manipulation of qualitative data (Ramazanoglu and Holland, 1992; Seidel *et al.*, 1988), although the size of our database rather stretched the capacities of the program in the case of the young women. The questionnaire data were analyzed with the use of SPSS.
7   See Holland *et al.*, 1991, 1992a, 1992b, forthcoming.
8   Further vulnerability is created for many young men in that they do not believe in, or agree with, the male model of sexuality by which they are judged. It is possible for both men and women to resist the social pressures of masculinity and femininity, but in practice few manage such resistance (for example, coming out as gay while still at school, or developing a positive female sexuality (Holland *et al.*, 1992a)). We do not have space to develop our data on the difficulties and possibilities of resistance here.
9   See Holland *et al.*, (1992a) for an appropriated female form of this instrumental model.
10   Daniel Wight found this response in his sample of 19-year-old men (personal communication). See also Wight, 1993 and forthcoming.
11   Kelly *et al.*, (1991, p. 7), in their study of child abuse reported by 1200 16-to-21-year-olds, found three cases where older women sexualized relationships with young men, but the young men did not experience these as victimizing. The same was true in the one case of female-on-male child sexual abuse reported in our data. See also Fromuth and Burkhart (1987).
12   There is a complex interplay of factors from which power can be derived — age, knowledge, gender, 'race' which can lead to a delicate balance of relational power. In this case the young man has focused on differential age as legitimizing a shift in the balance of gendered power.

References

ALLEN, I. (1987) *Education in Sex and Personal Relationships,* PSI Report No. 665.

BACK, L. (1993) 'Gendered Participation: Masculinity and Fieldwork in a South London Adolescent Community', in BELL, D., CAPLAN, P. and KARIM, W.J. (Eds) *Gendered Fields: Women, Men and Ethnography,* London, Routledge.

BOWIE, C. and FORD, N. (1989) 'Sexual Behaviour of Young People and the Risk of HIV Infection' *Journal of Epidemiology and Community Health,* vol. 43, no. 1, pp. 61 5.

BRITTAN, A. (1989) *Masculinity and Power,* Oxford, Blackwell.

BROD, H. (Ed.) (1987) *The Making of Masculinities,* Boston, Allen and Unwin.

CARRIGAN, T., CONNELL, R.W. and LEE, J. (1985) 'Toward a New Sociology of Masculinity', *Theory and Society,* vol. 14, no. 5, pp. 551 604.

CHAPMAN, R. and RUTHERFORD, J. (Eds) (1988) *Male Order: Unwrapping Masculinity,* London, Lawrence and Wishart.

CLATTERBAUGH, K. (1990) *Contemporary Perspectives on Masculinity: Men, Women and Politics in Modern Society,* Boulder, Colorado, Westview Press.

CURRIE, C. (1990) 'Young People in Independent Schools, Sexual Behaviour and AIDS'. In AGGLETON, P., DAVIES, P. and HART, G. (Eds) *AIDS: Individual, Cultural and Policy Dimensions,* London, Falmer Press.

DAVIES, P.M., HICKSON, F.C.I., WEATHERBURN, P. and HUNT, A.J. (1993) *Sex, Gay Men and AIDS,* London, Falmer Press.

FORD, N. (1991) *The Socio-Sexual Lifestyles of Young People in South West England,* Exeter, SWRHA/Institute of Population Studies.

FORD, N. and MORGAN, K. (1989) 'Heterosexual Lifestyles of Young People in an English City', *Journal of Population and Social Studies,* vol. 1, no. 2, pp. 167 85.

FROMUTH, M. and BURKHART, B. (1987) 'Childhood Sexual Victimisation among College Men: Definitional and Methodological Issues', *Violence and Victims,* vol. 2, no. 4, pp. 533–42.

HEARN, J. and MORGAN, D. (Eds) (1990) Men, Masculinities and Social Theory, London, Unwin Hyman.

HOLLAND, J. (1993) *Sexuality and Ethnicity: Variations in Young Women's Sexual Knowledge and Practice,* WRAP Paper 8, London, Tufnell Press.

HOLLAND, J. and RAMAZANOGLU, C. (forthcoming) 'Coming to Conclusions: Power and Interpretation in Researching Young Women's Sexuality', in PURVIS, J. and MAYNARD, M. (Eds) *Researching Women's Lives from a Feminist Perspective,* London, Falmer Press.

HOLLAND, J., RAMAZANOGLU, C., SCOTT, S., SHARPE, S. and THOMSON. R. (1991) 'Between Embarrassment and Trust: Young Women and the Diversity of Condom Use', in AGGLETON, P., DAVIES, P. and HART, G. (Eds) *AIDS: Responses, Interventions and Care,* London, Falmer Press.

HOLLAND, J., RAMAZANOGLU, C., SCOTT, S., SHARPE, S. and THOMSON, R. (1992a) 'Pressure, Resistance, Empowerment: Young Women and the Negotiation of Safer Sex', in AGGLETON, P., DAVIES, P. and HART, G. (Eds) *AIDS: Rights, Risk and Reason,* London, Falmer Press.

HOLLAND, J., RAMAZANOGLU, C., SHARPE, S. and THOMSON, R. (1992b) 'Pleasure, Pressure and Power: Some Contradictions of Gendered Sexuality' *Sociological Review,* vol. 40, no. 4, pp. 645–74.

HOLLAND, J., RAMAZANOGLU, C., SHARPE, S. and THOMSON, R. (forthcoming) 'Power and Desire: The Embodiment of Female Sexuality', *Feminist Review.*

HOLLWAY, W. (1981) '"I Just Wanted To Kill a Woman". Why? The Ripper and Male Sexuality', *Feminist Review,* no. 9, pp. 33–40.

HOLLWAY, W. (1984) 'Women's Power in Heterosexual Sex', *Women's Studies International Forum,* vol. 7, pp. 63–8.

KELLY, L., REGAN, L. and BURTON, S. (1991) *An Exploratory Study of the Prevalence of Sexual Abuse in a Sample of 16–21 year olds,* Child Abuse Studies Unit, Polytechnic of North London, 62–66 Ladbroke House, Highbury Grove, London N5 2AD.

KENT, V., DAVIES, M., DEVERELL, K. and GOTTESMAN, S. (1990) 'Social Interaction Routines Involved in Heterosexual Encounters: Prelude to First Intercourse', paper presented at the Fourth Conference on the Social Aspects of AIDS, London.

KIMMEL, M.S. (Ed.) (1987) *Changing Men: New Directions in Research on Men and Masculinity,* Newbury Park, California, Sage.

LEES, S. (1993) *Sugar and Spice: Sexuality and Adolescent girls,* London, Penguin.

LITEWKA, J. (1977) 'The Socialised Penis', in SNODGRASS, J. (Ed.) *For Men Against Sexism,* Albion, California, Times Change Press.

MORGAN, D. (1981) 'Men, Masculinity and the Process of Sociological Enquiry', in ROBERTS, H. (Ed.) *Doing Feminist Research,* London, Routledge and Kegan Paul.

NIX, L.M., PASTEUR, A.B. and SERVANCE, M.A. (1988) 'A Focus Group Study of Sexually Active Black Male Teenagers', *Adolescence,* vol. 23, no. 91, pp. 741–3.

RAMAZANOGLU, C. (1992) 'What Can You Do with a Man? Feminism and the Critical Appraisal of Masculinity', *Women's Studies International Forum,* vol. 15, no. 3, pp. 339 50.

RAMAZANOGLU, C. and HOLLAND, J. (1992) 'Using the Ethnograph as a Research Tool', paper given at conference, An Introduction to Computers in Qualitative Analysis, University of Southampton, January.

SEGAL, L. (1990) *Slow Motion,* London, Virago.

SEIDEL, J.V., KJOLSETH, R. and SEYMOUR, E. (1988) *The Ethnograph: A User's Guide,* Littleton, Colarado, Qualis Research Associates.

SEIDLER, V.J. (1989) *Rediscovering Masculinity: Reason, Language and Sexuality,* London, Routledge.

SEIDLER, V.J. (1991a) *Recreating Sexual Politics: Men, Feminism and Politics,* London, Routledge.

SEIDLER, V.J. (Ed.) (1991b) *The Achilles Heel Reader: Men, Sexual Politics and Socialism,* London, Routledge.

THOMSON, R. and SCOTT, S. (1991) *Learning about Sex: Young Women and the Social Construction of Sexual Identity,* London, Tufnell Press.

WIGHT, D. (1993) 'Constraints or Cognition: Factors Affecting Young Men's Practice of Safer Heterosexual Sex', in AGGLETON, P., DAVIES, P. and HART, G. (Eds) *AIDS: The Second Decade,* London, Falmer Press.

WIGHT, D. (forthcoming) 'Boys' Thoughts and Talk about Sex in a Working Class Locality of Glasgow', *Sociological Review.*

WOOD, J. (1987) 'Groping towards Sexism: Boys' Sex Talk', in WEINER, G. and ARNOT, M. (Eds) *Gender Under Scrutiny: New Inquiries in Education,* London: Unwin Hyman.

Section IV

Live Issues for a Feminist Agenda

Chapter 9

Feminists, Prostitutes and HIV

Kate Butcher

When HIV was first discovered to be sexually transmitted, prostitution became the focus of media attention. Images of women as dispensers of infection reappeared, reminiscent of Second World War VD campaigns. The public has always demanded scapegoats, and this held true for HIV. As usual, public attention fell on women involved in prostitution, and responsibility for infection became theirs by proxy 'as though they were acting on their own' (Morgan-Thomas, 1991). Untangling truth from untruth, a clear picture emerges of prostitutes themselves as only part of a larger cast of clients, managers, police and pimps. While health promotion and HIV prevention projects are increasingly acknowledging the need to include as many players in the field of prostitution as possible (Kinnell, 1989; Overs, 1991), it is now time to review how prostitutes and prostitution fit into the scenario of HIV/AIDS. Over a decade into the epidemic it is equally important to assess the role that feminism may have to play in the lives of millions of women across the world who are involved in the sex industry.

Towards a Definition of Prostitution

Definitions of prostitution, and the social and moral complexities with which such definitions engage, need first to be addressed. Women who sell sex commercially may choose to describe themselves in a variety of ways: as escorts, masseuses, working women, or simply as prostitutes. For the sake of expediency the term 'prostitution' will be used here, but as with any social labelling, it is crucial that the women in question are allowed to define themselves as they choose. The variety of terms reflect the diversity of work within the industry, but it is as well to note that defining any woman solely in terms of the work she performs obscures her other identities as an individual, a daughter, perhaps a sister, wife or mother. It is precisely this set of other identities which we should seek to restore.

Our understanding of this issue is profoundly influenced by particular historical, moral and cultural perspectives. The emphasis in the industrialized West, and to some extent in Asia, has been on 'professional' prostitutes, but studies in Africa reveal that the definition of prostitution is more complex than is generally assumed. As Sanders and Sambo point out, 'The majority of "prostitutes" in Africa cannot be categorized clearly and the term "prostitute" is not generally appropriate to the exchange of sexual services for money' (Sanders and Sambo, 1991). In Kenya the word 'Malaya' is used to describe 'some form of prostitution and other informal unions that involve not only exchange of sex for money but also provision of food and lodging' (Day, 1988). In Zimbabwe, 'the exchange of sex for money covers a broad range of arrangements. Many are not socially considered to be prostitution'. Divorcees or women separated from their husbands commonly only take up liaisons with other men where there is financial compensation, 'but none would consider herself a prostitute' (Bassett and Mhloyi, 1991). When considering HIV prevention, all women should have equal access to education, information and the means to protect themselves, regardless of their social label. Indeed, there is a strong argument that those who bear the greatest stigma are in need of more resources.

Gender and Power

At a time when women are beginning to demand equality with men, questions of power and gender are unavoidable. Maxine Ankrah writes from Uganda that 'the concept of maleness which hinges on the subordination of women must be exposed . . . the concept of "empowerment" may be viewed as a strategy to reinforce efforts of the African male to a new perception of his female partner — as an equal' (Ankrah, 1991). The juxtaposition of power and prostitution has a particular resonance, since it embraces so many variables of power imbalance: economic, fiscal, sexual and political.

Women are involved in prostitution throughout the world. Some have made a decision to work in the industry; some are coerced into it or sold into it. Whatever the story of an individual woman, invariably economics is a major theme. Women striving to be financially independent may find prostitution the only option open to them. For some young women in Britain, where the alternatives are either £5 a week pocket-money in care or £25 a week on state benefit, working in prostitution may appear to be the only way to survive in a society where status revolves around material goods and designer labels. For women with children to support the alternatives are often similar. In other parts of the world, women do not have access even to these inadequate options. In India in 1990, there was a move to encourage women out of prostitution by offering them a lump sum equivalent to £50. For women earning up to the equivalent of £15 a day, the likelihood of this approach succeeding was minimal (Anonymous, 1990).

Perceiving all women who work in prostitution as victims belies the strength of those for whom it is a positive choice, or lucrative work. Discouraging prostitution is not automatically a helpful response, although there are clearly circumstances — such as child prostitution — where there is a moral obligation to protect an individual from harm by removing her from this line of work. The decision to do so is fraught with problems however — at what point, for example, does a young woman no longer need 'protection' from prostitution? 'Third party sexual abuse' is the term used in this country in relation to the use of young women under the age of consent in the sex industry. Does reaching the legal age of consent mean that a young woman is any more in control of her experience? While the International Congress for Prostitutes' Rights recognizes that prostitution is 'adult work', at what point do young women in different cultures become adult?

HIV, AIDS and Prostitution

As far as HIV is concerned, the most immediate necessity is to reduce the risk for women involved in prostitution. This process is inextricably linked to the legal position of prostitutes and their work in any given country. Current debates in the West revolve around state regulation, giving little thought to the alternative of decriminalizing prostitution itself. If women were no longer criminalized for selling sex, the stigma attached to their work might eventually diminish, and prostitutes would be able to work without fear of recrimination and legal penalty. Supporting greater self-determination for all women means lobbying for decriminalization, giving prostitutes equal status with other self-employed groups in their respective countries.

Current laws in the UK not only make the job of prostitutes more dangerous, but keep women ensnared in the trap of fines and often subjugation to a pimp. If kerbcrawling is illegal, women do not have time to determine whether or not a prospective partner is safe (Lopez

Jones, 1990). Heavy policing serves to move women away from areas where they may have established support networks to unknown territory where they are more vulnerable. The murder of prostitute women is not an uncommon occurrence. Prostitution itself is not illegal. However, it is illegal to live off 'immoral earnings', and for two or more prostitutes to live and work together, laws which successfully disempower prostitute women, debarring them from the relative safety of working collectively, and making them constantly vulnerable to arrest.

In the light of HIV, the attitude of the judiciary to condom use is unhelpful to say the least. While some courts continue to use the possession of condoms as evidence against women for soliciting (English Collective of Prostitutes, 1991), the judge in a recent rape trial 'praised a rapist for wearing a condom, claiming that he had acted with kindness and consideration' (*Guardian,* 1991). At a time when public health campaigns urge us to 'act responsibly', the law is clearly not acting *fairly* on behalf of women.

The legal undermining of women's rights occurs elsewhere in the world. In 1990 in Thailand a green card system was introduced for prostitutes testing negative for HIV antibodies, so that clients could take their pleasures without the inconvenience of latex (Smith, 1990). Not only does this endanger the livelihood of those women who use condoms in their work, it also endangers their lives. The main source of income for the Philippines, including Filipino 'hospitality women', is work derived from the presence of US army bases (Tan *et al.,* 1989). Until recently Philippine law mandated the HIV testing of long-term visitors 'with the exception of US military personnel' (Scott, 1992).

Risk and Safety

Most HIV/AIDS projects in the West which have concentrated on 'professional' prostitution have concluded that women almost always use condoms at work, and there is more risk of prostitute women themselves acquiring HIV infection within their non-paying sexual relationships than there is of paying clients becoming infected (Kinnell, 1989). It has been said elsewhere that in general the equations 'work = sex with a condom' and 'pleasure = sex without a condom' hold good (Kinnell, 1989). The condom is more than protection against disease, it is a physical barrier, a metaphor of exclusion for the woman at work, keeping the punter symbolically as far away as possible. Work with prostitutes needs to go further than the simple provision of condoms. Priscilla Alexander's CAL-PEP project pioneers educational initiatives involving the prostitutes themselves in recognition of their skill as sex workers and their potential as AIDS educators (Alexander, 1988).

Involving prostitutes in discussions about how to protect their health *outside* work is essential. Prostitute women often do not want to use condoms at home because it is reminiscent of work. In addition, the rarely challenged culture of heterosexual sex and its inevitable identification with penetration makes discussion of safer sexual alternatives difficult. It has also been suggested that the higher up the ladder of prostitution a woman works, the more at risk she is likely to be (Kinnell, 1989). Clients at the highest level are paying for the fantasy that their 'girls' are available exclusively to them (Day, 1988; Kinnell, 1989). Using condoms introduces the idea of multiple partners and therefore shatters the illusion which is being bought.

Since the major risk of infection is through heterosexual sex, and since in the West women appear to be more vulnerable than men to heterosexual transmission, understanding the culture of heterosex and especially the centrality of the penis (Miles, 1989) is crucial to protecting women from the virus. The whole concept of romantic love and love-making evolved from the days of mediaeval chivalry, which developed and consolidated the idea of women as passive creatures, damsels in distress. This concept remains embedded in current popular thought throughout the West and to a large extent determines what options we believe to be available. As Tamsin Wilton suggests, 'A systematic deconstruction of masculinity is . . . central . . . to radical AIDS discourse' (Wilton, 1990). Kathryn Caravano adds that 'efforts to prevent the spread of AIDS to women must therefore focus on empowerment, on the repossession by women of our bodies' (Caravano, 1991). According to Helen Haste, 'challenging the metaphors of gender is part of a wider contemporary challenge to some of the cherished metaphors by which we categorise, dichotomise and explain our world' (Haste, 1992). Discussion on how to make this challenge effective is vital to the success of *all* heterosexual women in being able to practise safer sex with men and thereby to protect their health. In many countries where women working in the sex industry are organizing collectively, this discussion is beginning to take place. Groups such as Empower in Bangkok, Coyote in California and the English Collective of Prostitutes in London demonstrate that prostitutes are joining together to find strength in collaboration, and protecting themselves from HIV is high on the agenda.

Complex Problems – A Feminist Solution?

There are additional dimensions to the debate around sexual power. In some cases young girls from 12 to 16 years of age work as prostitutes. They often have a poor understanding of their health needs in general and their sexual health in particular, and are therefore less likely to take steps to protect themselves. Pregnancy is still considered the most immediate problem. This lack of knowledge may increase younger women's vulnerability, since 'most clients are not concerned with protecting others' (Leonard, 1990).

Another dimension which cannot be overlooked is the part played in prostitution by drug use. Once addictive drugs — including alcohol — enter the picture, levels of protection drop (Plant, 1990). In some areas there is a correlation between drug use and prostitution (Philpot *et al.*, 1988; Sattaur, 1991; Plant, 1990). Violence is clearly an issue: if a client is under the influence of alcohol or narcotics the likelihood of violence is increased and the degree of control the prostitute has over the encounter diminishes. In terms of immediate survival, 'violence is a greater threat (than HIV)' (Herrell, 1991).

If these are some of the dynamics of the question of power and prostitution, what role may feminism play? Certainly the subject of prostitution has met with an ambivalent response from feminists for some years. The International Committee for Prostitutes' Rights voiced the feeling that whether or not women chose to work in the industry, whether they enjoyed it or loathed it, they felt an overwhelming sense of exclusion and rejection from feminists (Pheterson, 1990). At the second World Whores' Congress held in Brussels in 1986 a statement on prostitution and feminism was drawn up, outlining nine basic rights. These included the rights of women to live free from stigma, to have equal access to a full range of employment and educational alternatives including prostitution, to financial autonomy and self-determination. The Congress made a clear call for an alliance of *all* women. In the era of HIV/AIDS, with endless struggles for funding and in the face of attempts to divide and rule, it is more vital than ever that women work together to prevent the spread of HIV and the stigma that accompanies it.

Feminists across the world have a major role to play in protecting the lives and health of prostitute women. These women are as diverse a group as any other, with equally complex lives. They may be black or white, upper-class or working-class, wealthy or poor, lesbian or heterosexual. It is vital that we recognize our points of commonality rather than focusing on difference, so that prostitute and non-prostitute women can work together to combat HIV infection and the stigma attached to it.

We can encourage projects working with prostitution to broaden their focus to include all the players, thereby making it clear that prostitutes themselves can only shoulder part of the responsibility. This will serve to lay a fair share of responsibility at the feet of sexually active heterosexual men. Any work focusing on sexual health within the community should actively seek the involvement of local prostitutes, recognizing their skills and experience in this area. Feminists should also consider their position in relation to the decriminalization of prostitution as an integral part of the struggle to restore self-determination to all women, including those working as prostitutes. All women would reap the benefits of this as a strategy for achieving wider recognition of our collective rights. 'When any woman can walk the streets at night . . . without running the risk of being branded a whore, arrested for street walking or raped . . . we will know that the theory of women's liberation from male violence has been translated into fact' (Roberts, 1992).

References

ALEXANDER, PRISCILLA (1988) CAL-PEP, P.O. Box 6297, San Francisco, CA 94010-6297.

ANKRAH, E. MAXINE (1991) 'AIDS and the Social Side of Health', *Social Science and Medicine*, vol. 32, no. 9, pp. 967-80.

ANONYMOUS (1990) 'India: Prostitutes and the Spread of AIDS', *Lancet*, vol. 335, 2 June, p. 1332.

BASSETT, MARY T. and MHLOYI, MARVELLOUS (1991) 'Women and AIDS in Zimbabwe: The Making of an Epidemic', *International Journal of Health Services*, vol. 21, no. 1, pp. 143-56.

CARAVANO, KATHRYN (1991) 'More than Mothers and Whores: Redefining the AIDS Prevention Needs of Women', *International Journal of Health Services*, vol. 21, no. 1, pp. 131-42.

DALY, MARY (1979) *Gyn/Ecology: The Meta Ethics of Radical Feminism*, London, Women's Press.

DAY, SOPHIE (1988) 'Prostitute Women and AIDS: Anthropology', *AIDS*, vol. 2, no. 6, pp. 421-8.

ENGLISH COLLECTIVE OF PROSTITUTES (1991) 'Appeal for Letters to the Home Secretary', Unpublished Letter, 25 September.

GUARDIAN (1991) 'Judge Praises Rapist', 12 April.

HASTE, HELEN (1992) 'Splitting Images: Sex and Science', *New Scientist*, 15 February.

HERRELL, RICHARD K. (1991) 'HIV/AIDS Research and the Social Sciences' Conference Report, *Current Anthropology*, vol. 32, no. 2, April.

JOCHELSON, K., MOTHIBELI, M. and LEGER, J.P. (1991) 'Human Immunodeficiency Virus and Migrant Labor in South Africa, *International Journal of Health Services*, vol. 21, no. 1, pp. 157-73.

KINNELL, HILARY (1989) 'Prostitutes, Their Clients and Risks of HIV Infection', Occasional Paper, Dept. Public Health Medicine, C.B.H.A., Vincent Drive, Edgbaston, BIRMINGHAM B15 2TZ.

KRIEGER, NANCY and MARGO, GLEN (1991) 'Women and AIDS: Introduction', *International Journal of Health Services,* vol. 21, no. 1, pp. 127–30.

LEONARD, T. (1990) 'Male Clients of Female Street Prostitutes', *Medical Anthropology Quarterly,* vol. 4, no. 1, pp. 41–5.

LOPEZ JONES, NINA (1990) 'Prostitutes: Guilty Until Proven Innocent', *New Law Journal,* 11 May.

MILES, ROSALIND (1989) *A Woman's History of the World,* London, Paladin.

MORGAN-THOMAS, RUTH (1991) 'The Sex Industry', *AIDS Action,* issue 15 (September).

OVERS, C. (1991) 'How to Sell Safer Sex', *AIDS Action,* issue 15 (September).

PADIAN, NANCY (1988) 'Prostitute Women and AIDS: Epidemiology', *AIDS,* vol. 2, no. 6, pp. 413–18.

PHETERSON, GAIL (1990) *A Vindication of Whores' Rights,* Seal Press.

PHILPOT, C.R., HARCOURT, C., EDWARDS, J. and GREALIS, A. (1988) 'Human Immunodeficiency Virus and Female Prostitutes', *Genitourinary Medicine,* vol. 64, pp. 193–7.

PLANT, MARTIN A. (Ed.) (1990) *Aids, Drugs and Prostitution,* London, Routledge.

ROBERTS, N. (1992) 'The Whore Stigma', *Cosmopolitan,* May.

SANDERS, DAVID and SAMBO, ABDULRAHMAN (1991) 'AIDS in Africa: The Implications of Economic Recession and Structural Adjustment', *Health Policy and Planning,* vol. 6, no. 2, pp. 157–65.

SATTAUR, OMAR (1991) 'India Wakes Up To AIDS', *New Scientist,* 2 November.

SCOTT, PETER (Ed.) (1992) *National AIDS Manual,* London, NAM Publications (Topics Section F4-4).

SMITH, D. (1990) 'Green Cards for Thai Sex Workers', *World AIDS,* July, p. 3.

TAN, MICHAEL, DE LEON, ADUL, STOLTZFUS, BRENDA and O'DONNELL, CINDY (1989) 'AIDS as a Political Issue: Working with the Sexually Prostituted in the Philippines', *Community Development Journal,* vol. 24, no. 3, pp. 186–93.

WILSON, D., CHIRARO, P., LAVELLE, S. and MUTERO, C. (1989) 'Sex Worker, Client Sex Behaviour and Condom Use in Harare, Zimbabwe, *AIDS Care,* vol. 1, no. 3, pp. 269–80.

WILTON, TAMSIN (1990) 'Condoms, Coercion and Control: Heterosexuality and the Limits to HIV/AIDS Education', paper presented at Fourth Conference on Social Aspects of AIDS.

Chapter 10

Inclusions and Exclusions: Lesbians, HIV and AIDS

Diane Richardson

What Have HIV and AIDS Got To Do With Lesbians?

To many people the answer to this question is easy: very little. The general assumption seems to be that lesbians as a group are not at risk. Lesbians don't get AIDS, so what's it got to do with them? Set against this view has been the stereotyping of AIDS as a 'gay disease', which in the past has led to lesbians being labelled as 'high-risk'. In some countries, for example, lesbians have been refused as blood donors on the grounds of their 'homosexuality'. Thus, lesbians are both implicated in popular conceptions of AIDS which link homosexuality and disease and neglected in the health care system's response to AIDS. They are simultaneously included and excluded in the AIDS discourse, upon which research, AIDS education and health care have been based.

Questions of difference and exclusion are central to the position of lesbians in media and medical constructions of AIDS and HIV. Lesbians are largely absent from the literature on AIDS, AIDS education campaigns usually ignore us, we are left out of public discussions about AIDS and HIV, and research is virtually non-existent. This is perhaps hardly surprising given that lesbians are rendered invisible in many aspects of life. More specifically, however, there exists a general lack of recognition of lesbian health issues, in particular the position of lesbians as receivers of health care (see Burns, 1992; Stern, 1993).

Even within the gay community the relevance of the AIDS crisis to lesbians is often not acknowledged. Indeed, some gay men are highly critical of lesbians wanting to discuss how AIDS and HIV affect them, and see it as lesbians jumping on the bandwagon or, as some have put it, having 'virus envy' (O'Sullivan and Parmar, 1992). It is also true that many lesbians do not see AIDS or HIV as an issue affecting them. For example, Sheffield AIDS education project entitled their leaflet for lesbians 'Lesbians, HIV and AIDS: Are You Serious?' on the basis of the comments made by lesbians themselves. Surprise is not the only reaction. Sometimes discussion of AIDS/HIV has led to angry debates, with lesbians who raise the subject of lesbians and safer sex being accused of being hysterical or, worse still, of frightening other lesbians unnecessarily.

Why is this? Why do such reactions occur? One possible explanation is that very few lesbians, at present, know other lesbians who are HIV-infected, so the issues may feel more theoretical, more at a distance than they do for gay men. Clearly this is likely to change as more lesbians are identified as being HIV-positive or having AIDS. It is also significant that IV drug use, having sex with men (whether for payment or not), even talking about the kinds of sex women have together, are often taboo issues within lesbian communities, which complicates the whole issue of discussing lesbians, HIV and AIDS.

The lack of coverage of lesbians and AIDS has also encouraged the 'Are You Serious?' attitude among lesbians. The health care system is designed for and administered by a predominantly heterosexual population, resulting in a general lack of recognition of lesbian health issues. This lack of knowledge has stimulated women's research into health issues relevant to themselves as lesbians and the publication of handbooks such as *Alive and Well: A Lesbian Health Guide* (Hepburn and Gutierrez, 1988) and *Lesbian Health Matters* (O'Donnell *et a.,* 1980). Similarly, medical research and publications are extremely deficient in information concerning health issues specific to lesbians. There is relatively little known, for example, about if and how women sexually transmit certain infections to each other. It is therefore not surprising that, despite an enormous and ever increasing literature on AIDS and HIV, little attention has been paid to the specific ways in which AIDS/HIV affects lesbians.

There are only a handful of studies that have looked at risk behaviour among lesbians. As with other social groups, the main risk activities for HIV infection are sharing equipment to inject drugs and (especially unprotected) vaginal or anal intercourse with a man. Lesbians may also be at risk of infection through donor insemination. (For a more detailed discussion of AIDS and donor insemination see Richardson, 1993.)

According to various surveys many lesbians occasionally have sex with men or have done so in the recent past. One US study reported that 79 per cent of lesbians interviewed had experienced vaginal intercourse at some point in their life, and approximately one in ten were still having sex with men (Saghir and Robins, 1973). In a recent survey of sexual behaviour in Britain, 54% of the women who said they had had a female sexual partner in the previous two years had had sex with a man in the same period (Wellings *et al.*, 1994).

We know less about the extent of IV drug use and needle sharing within lesbian communities. Among the lesbians with AIDS reported by the CDC in the US, most are assumed to have acquired HIV through risk practices associated with IV drug use (though see comments below on the construction of AIDS figures). In San Francisco, as part of the Urban Health Study, the Lesbian AIDS Project is studying the rate of infection among (self-identified) lesbian IV drug users. Similarly, an Italian study interviewed 342 'homo/bisexual' women to analyze the potential for HIV transmission and to evaluate the perception of HIV infection among lesbians and bisexual women (Sasse *et al.*, 1992). Seven women were reported to be HIV-positive, of whom six said that they believed they had been infected through sharing equipment to inject drugs and one through sexual intercourse with a man. The results of the study suggest that there may be a significant proportion of bisexual behaviour and injecting drug use among some groups of lesbians. One in ten of the women interviewed said they had injected drugs at some point in their life and most of these said they had shared equipment to do so. Interestingly, 26 per cent of the sample reported having had an HIV test.

Although woman-to-woman sexual transmission of HIV appears to be extremely rare, the issue is still largely unexamined in the literature. Very few cases of possible female-to-female transmission have, so far, been reported in the literature (Sabatini *et al.*, 1984; Marmor *et al.*, 1986; Monzon and Capellan, 1987; Perry *et al.*, 1989). Anecdotally however, there have been claims that women have sexually transmitted HIV to each other (Solomon, 1992). In addition, there is at least one documented case of a man acquiring HIV through cunnilingus (Spitzer and Weiner, 1989).

The assumption that lesbians are not at risk of HIV infection and/or affected by AIDS is also reinforced by the lack of epidemiological data. Unlike reports of male cases, government statistics rarely classify cases of AIDS or HIV infection in women according to whether they are heterosexual, bisexual or lesbian. In the United States, the Centers for Disease Control (CDC) has provided some information on lesbians and AIDS. They analyzed US surveillance data for the 9,717 cases of AIDS in women reported between June 1980 and September 1989. The women were grouped either as lesbian (reporting sex only with female partners since 1977), bisexual (reporting sex with both male and female partners since 1977), or heterosexual (reporting sex with only male partners since 1977). Among the seventy-nine women who were classified as lesbian, seventy-five were reported to have acquired HIV infection via risk practices associated with intravenous drug use. The other four became infected following a blood transfusion. Among the 103 women defined as bisexual, 79 per cent were intravenous drug users, 16 per cent had male sexual partners who were either HIV-positive or at increased risk of infection, and 4 per cent had histories of blood transfusion (Chu *et al.*, 1990).

Estimates of the number of lesbians in the United States who are HIV-infected tend to be in the low hundreds (Schneider, 1992), but no one really knows how many lesbians are infected with HIV or have AIDS in the US or anywhere else. The CDC data should not be regarded as an accurate record of lesbians with AIDS; rather, the figures represent those women who were known by the CDC to have had sex with other women. Women were not asked if they had sex with other women and if they did not define themselves otherwise they would be presumed heterosexual (Leonard, 1990). Also, the CDC's definition of a lesbian as a woman who has reported having had sexual relations *exclusively* with women since 1977 means that if a lesbian had sex with a man, maybe only once or twice, she is no longer counted as a lesbian because of it.

It is also important to remember that the CDC, like other surveillance organizations, uses a hierarchy of categories of risk for exposure to HIV: intravenous drug use, receipt of blood products, heterosexual contact with a partner having HIV infection or a specified risk for infection, and no identified risk. (Because no specific category exists for female-to-female exposure, reports of such transmission would fall into the latter category.) What this means in practice is that women with multiple risks are assigned to only one exposure category, unlike men who now may be placed into multiple risk categories (e.g. gay male IVDU). In other words, if a lesbian uses or used IV drugs, even if she never shared needles, or if she has had sex with a man since 1977, it is likely that she would be put under the category IVDU or, in the latter case, heterosexual contact, even if her female partner(s) were HIV-infected or considered to be at risk for infection. The possibility of woman-to-woman transmission would be ignored.

What are the implications of this lack of information? By thinking AIDS is an issue which does not affect them, some lesbians may be putting themselves at risk of HIV infection. Equally, some lesbians who are ill-informed may be worrying unnecessarily about HIV infection or AIDS. Risk of HIV infection is created by certain kinds of behaviour, not by social group or sexual identity. Despite this, many people still think about AIDS as affecting certain 'risk groups'; and lesbians, it is often assumed, are not, as a group, at risk. This perception has important implications for the prevention of transmission of HIV. On a theoretical level, it also prompts a number of questions about the relationship between sexual conduct and sexual identity, and about the important differences between the category 'lesbian' and the category 'gay' or 'homosexual' (see also Boston Lesbian Psychologies Collective, 1987).

The invisibility of lesbians in the AIDS crisis is important for other reasons. It tells us, for instance, a great deal about the way lesbians are defined. It begs the question 'What is a lesbian?'. Presumably, a lesbian is someone who does not and never will inject drugs or share needles, someone who does not and will not have sex with men, someone who does not get sexually abused or raped, and who does not try to get pregnant. The dominant construction of lesbians as a social group defined by its sexuality means that the traditional perception of lesbians is as women who sexually desire and have sex with other women and little else. This is vitally important to understanding resistance to demands for AIDS/HIV education for lesbians. The construction of lesbians as essentially sexual, in conjunction with the fact that woman-to-woman transmission appears to be extremely rare, leads many to conclude that lesbians are neither at risk nor in need of information about risk. However, as Sue O'Sullivan and Pratibha Parmar point out, 'The recognition that positive lesbians exist challenges old fixed notions of lesbian identity' (O'Sullivan and Parmar, 1992, p. 49). It also raises issues about what constitutes lesbian sex.

The general opinion seems to be that belonging to the category 'lesbian' automatically means that your sexual practices do not transmit HIV. This reflects, in part, the phallocentric view of 'sex' as penis in vagina, which restricts the categorization of other activities as 'sexual'. (The frequent absence of lesbianism as a sexual practice in most AIDS education material is a good example of the denial of lesbian sexuality.) And if lesbian sex is not 'sex' then presumably HIV and other sexually transmitted infections are not an issue. In other words, dominant discourses of sex render 'sex between women as more invisible, but also more harmless' (Richardson, 1992).

Is lesbian sex, by definition, safe? Whilst sex between women involves a lower range of risks than vaginal or anal intercourse, there are still questions to be asked about lesbian sexuality and the possible risks of certain activities, especially if risk (and safety) are defined in broader terms than simply transmission of HIV (see pp. 152–53). Although it is unclear whether the presence of HIV in menstrual blood, vaginal and cervical secretions means that it can be passed on during sex from one woman to another, certain other sexually transmitted infections such as herpes, thrush and chlamydia, can be so passed on. Also, as women and as lesbians we may argue that sex has never been safe in a society that encourages sexual violence towards women, is anti-lesbian and attempts to deny women sexual autonomy. Most researchers and health educators have failed to address these issues, although some writers have outlined safer sex guidelines for lesbians in their work (e.g. Patton and Kelly, 1987; Richardson, 1989; O'Sullivan and Parmar, 1992). Recognition of these concerns may influence AIDS/HIV policy-making more generally, particularly in relation to safer sex campaigns given that the dominant construction of safer sex within these campaigns has been the correct use of condoms.

The safer sex campaigns that have been aimed at lesbians have tended to be centred around the risks of oral sex and the need for protection by dental dams (or a condom cut in two). In addition, the risks of sharing sex 'toys' have been highlighted. Interestingly, AIDS and HIV infection health education programmes aimed at heterosexual couples have not advised the use of dental dams during cunnilingus. In Britain a challenge to this emphasis on the risks of oral sex was provided, in 1992, by the controversial Terrence Higgins Trust advertising campaign aimed at informing lesbians on the relative risks of HIV infection in lesbian sex. The campaign claimed that lesbians are at 'very low risk in oral sex' and that therefore they should 'ditch those dental dams'. In the absence of research on whether or not HIV can be sexually transmitted from woman to woman, some lesbians reacted angrily to the THT campaign, claiming that it was irresponsible and would only serve to reinforce the assumption that lesbians, as a group, are not at risk.

Such debates have wider implications for lesbians beyond HIV and AIDS. For instance, for a variety of reasons (see Richardson, 1992) there has been a certain reluctance within the lesbian community to talk about desires and sexual practices. Ironically, the lack of certainty around the possibility of sexual transmission of HIV from one woman to another has created opportunities to talk more generally about negotiating sex, with safer sex as the starting point. AIDS has provided a context in which we are allowed to talk about sex, as have, in a different way, debates around sadomasochism. But irrespective of whether or not we can transmit HIV through sex with another woman, there are other reasons why we should be concerned about and involved in the politics of AIDS and HIV.

What Have Been the Effects of HIV and AIDS on Lesbians?

AIDS has impacted on lesbian communities in a number of ways, affecting lesbians who are at risk of HIV infection or are worried that they may have been in the past, lesbians who are HIV-positive or have AIDS, lesbians who are involved in AIDS work or in AIDS organizing as political activists, lesbians who are involved in caring for people with AIDS or HIV-related illness, and lesbians who have friends and family with HIV infection or AIDS. Also, because of the possible risks associated with self-insemination with donated sperm, the reproductive choices for lesbians have been affected. This is compounded by the fact that, in Britain, the introduction of stronger medical and legal control over donor insemination, with the passing of the 1990 Human Fertilisation and Embryology Act, has made it more difficult for lesbians to be inseminated through a clinic using sperm from screened donors. HIV/AIDS also highlights the need to address certain issues in the lesbian community, for example IV drug use.

For most lesbians, however, the main impact of AIDS has been the strengthening of social stereotypes and prejudices against lesbians as a group as a result of the way AIDS has been socially constructed. Of particular relevance is the way in which AIDS has revitalized the 'popular' association between certain forms of sexual behaviour/sexual relations and moral/physical health; especially the association between 'homosexuality' and disease (Patton, 1985). The categorization of lesbians together with gay men is clearly relevant here.

Increased anti-lesbian and anti-gay hostility and discrimination as a result of the ignorance and hysteria that has surrounded AIDS can affect lesbians in a variety of ways (Schneider, 1992). Many lesbians have been insulted and threatened. In some countries the rights of lesbians have been affected in areas of housing, employment and insurance cover, as well as access to and custody of their children. For example, in one case reported in the United States, a lesbian mother was denied visitation rights because of the judge's fear that she might give her children AIDS (Richardson, 1989).

More generally, AIDS has stimulated public debate on sexuality, sexual practice and sexual values which has prompted and/or encouraged attempts to impose new forms of social control over sexuality. These affect lesbians as well as other groups. A good example of this in Britain was Section 28 of the Local Government Act 1988, which makes it illegal for a local authority to intentionally 'promote' homosexuality and forbids the teaching of the 'acceptability of homosexuality as a pretended family relationship' (for a discussion see Stacey, 1991). We have since witnessed other attempts at discrimination in law, such as making it illegal for fertility clinics to offer lesbians artificial insemination. Although such attempts failed, Section 13 (5) of the Human Fertilisation and Embryology Act (1990) nevertheless states that 'a woman shall not be provided with treatment services unless account has been taken of the welfare of any child who may be born as a result of the treatment (including the need of that child for a father)'. As I have suggested above, it is hard to see how such a clause will not work against lesbians' insemination choices, which have already been affected because of HIV and AIDS.

The possible health implications of these trends are clearly worrying, not least because policies like these reinforce meanings of lesbianism that are highly negative. In a more general sense, however, lesbians may benefit from the fact that we are in the midst of a major challenge to ideas about sexuality because of HIV and AIDS. Most safer sex guidelines suggest, if sometimes rather apologetically, alternatives to intercourse, and this may help broaden notions of what 'sex' is. More importantly, from a lesbian point of view it may help to validate sex that does not involve a penis. Perhaps this means that in future we will be spared the age-old question: 'But what do you do?' which, when translated, means 'without a penis what can you do?'

What Are the Main Needs of Lesbians with Regard to HIV and AIDS?

One of the main needs that lesbians have in relation to HIV and AIDS is the need for information. Very few AIDS education efforts have been targeted at lesbians. We have hundreds of different brochures aimed at gay men, and expensive, glossy mass media campaigns aimed at heterosexuals (especially heterosexual women), yet what is there for lesbians? A leaflet if we are lucky. Many AIDS organizations, including some gay AIDS organizations, still have nothing to offer specifically for lesbians. This is all the more important where myths continue to exist that lesbians don't become HIV-infected or develop AIDS, and where public information campaigns can seem irrelevant. Being told repeatedly that the key to safer sex is 'Always Use A Condom' may not seem the most useful of advice to many lesbians (although I am not suggesting that condoms have no role in woman-to-woman sex). We also need to recognize that racism as well as heterosexism has informed the HIV and AIDS debate, and that black lesbians and gay men will have their own specific needs in relation to the provision of services and education.

In addition to a lack of information, lesbians also lack support services around HIV and AIDS. Lesbians are likely to have needs that differ from those of others who are HIV-infected or have AIDS, yet practically no services have been developed to specifically address them. Few support groups currently exist for women who have HIV infection or AIDS, let alone lesbian groups. If non-lesbian women with HIV infection or AIDS have found themselves isolated, then lesbians have even more so.

There are wider issues here for how the lesbian and gay community responds to AIDS. If other lesbians regard AIDS as irrelevant, this can only increase the sense of isolation lesbians with HIV or AIDS may feel. Similarly, in the gay community there has been a lack of interest in creating and supporting necessary services. This raises important questions about what AIDS organizations, and gay AIDS organizations in particular, should be doing. Should they be providing such services, or should these be provided by lesbian organizations? The argument for specialist lesbian services is a powerful one, but are lesbians likely to be in as powerful positions as gay men in obtaining AIDS/HIV funding?

This raises the question of how far we share common interests and political goals. To what extent do our interests as lesbians and gay men overlap? Many of the issues HIV and AIDS raises for women are different to the issues raised for men, most obviously in relation to reproduction, with the possibility that a woman with HIV may pass the virus on to the foetus. In terms of policy-making, serious questions are raised about protecting women's reproductive rights — both the rights of HIV-positive women to have children if they want them and access to abortion if they decide to terminate the pregnancy (Richardson, 1993).

Lesbians with HIV or AIDS have other needs which they are more likely to share with other women; for instance, women with AIDS are particularly likely to have housing difficulties, especially if they have dependant children, in which case there are also issues of childcare, including fostering and adoption, to consider. How often do AIDS/HIV policies address the needs of mothers and their children? There are other issues too; because, in general, women earn less than men, they are often more susceptible to the financial hardships which AIDS/HIV can bring.

In many respects, then, AIDS/HIV has a very different significance for lesbians than for gay men. It is not only a case of fewer numbers, that women with HIV infection have access to very limited services, that many housing programmes for people with AIDS are not designed for people with dependent children, that women find it hard to get on treatment and drug trials, that there is very little research on HIV-related infections in women. It is also about who gets the money, who makes the policy decisions, and who gets prioritized. Most of the medical literature concentrates on women as transmittors of HIV. The concern, overwhelmingly, is not about women and their health but about protecting the health of (heterosexual) men and children.

What Strategies Should We Adopt?

What we share as lesbians and gay men, of course, albeit to varying extents and in differing forms, is the experience of heterosexism and, related to that, certain aspects of AIDS discrimination. There is an AIDS double standard in which women, prostitutes, IV drug users, gay men and lesbians share in the public mind the category 'guilty'. It would seem that 'when women or gay/bisexual men get AIDS it is their fault, but if heterosexual men come down with the disease, it is the fault of women and gay/bisexual men'. (Alexander, 1988). To quote that well-known expert on lesbian affairs, Martina Navratilova, criticising the double standards that soon became apparent in the public response to the American basketball star Magic Johnson's announcement that he was HIV-positive and had contracted the virus through sexual intercourse with one of the hundreds of women he claimed to have had sex with,

> If I had the HIV virus would people be understanding? No, because they would say I'm gay, I had it coming . . . If it had happened to a heterosexual woman who had been with a hundred or two hundred men, they would call her a whore and a slut. (*Guardian,* 10 December 1991).

The question of how far we have interests in common is an important one. Lesbians have not only questioned the relevance of HIV and AIDS for lesbians, but the political desirability of getting involved in AIDS work in organizations which tend to be dominated by men and where policies often reflect men's interests and neglect women's. Elsewhere in this volume I have discussed lesbian/feminist politics and AIDS work in more detail (see pp. 44–45). Suffice it to say here, that whilst it is understandable and necessary that many services and organizations have been set up as a response to gay men's needs, we need to ask whether those services and organizations are prepared and willing to change to reflect the needs of other groups, in this case lesbians, or whether we should develop new services specific to our own needs?

What we need to bear in mind is that if we are to work together it will mean a commitment to understanding our different concerns. Often the question of unity is presented as a problem that lesbians have rather than relating to the way many AIDS organizations operate. To work together is not simply a question of saying, 'I'm happy if lesbians get involved in HIV and AIDS work'; our concerns, our differences, must be recognized, and policies, structures, and ways of working may need to change. Gay men and AIDS service providers might, for instance, learn a lot from the experiences of lesbians who have worked in the women's health movement. Equally, they may feel that lesbians working in HIV and AIDS are taking up valuable resources at a time when governments are failing to adequately fund health education services for gay men, who are the main group affected in the developed world.

It is essential that differences within lesbian and gay communities are debated, and that means debating issues of race and class as well as gender. However, these debates cannot merely be about identifying common issues that we share in relation to sexuality and health care, but must include a more fundamental analysis of the relationship between gender and sexuality and gender and health care. As lesbians we must do this now so that we can decide how, and in what ways, we wish to organize.

References

ALEXANDER, PRISCILLA (1988) 'Prostitutes Are Being Scapegoated for Heterosexual AIDS', in DELACOSTE, FRÉDÉRIQUE and ALEXANDER, PRISCILLA (Eds) *Sex Work*, London, Virago.

BOSTON LESBIAN PSYCHOLOGIES COLLECTIVE (Eds) (1987) *Lesbian Psychologies: Explorations and Challenges*, Urbana and Chicago, University of Illinois Press.

BURNS, JAN (1992) 'The Psychology of Lesbian Health Care', in NICOLSON, PAULA and USSHER, JANE (Eds) *The Psychology of Women's Health and Health Care*, London, Macmillan, pp. 225–48.

CHU, SUSAN, Y., BUEHLER, JAMES W., FLEMING, PATRICIA L. and BERKELMAN, RUTH L. (1990) 'Epidemiology of Reported Cases of AIDS in Lesbians, United States 1989-89', *American Journal of Public Health*, 80 (11), pp. 1380–1.

HEPBURN, CUCA and GUTIERREZ, BONNIE (1988) *Alive and Well: A Lesbian Health Guide*, New York, The Crossing Press.

LEONARD, ZOE (1990) 'Lesbians in the AIDS Crisis', in THE ACT UP/NEW YORK WOMEN AND AIDS BOOK GROUP *Women, AIDS, and Activism*, Boston, South End Press.

MARMOR, M., WEISS, L.R., LYDEN, M. *et al.* (1986) 'Possible Female to Female Transition of Human Immunodeficiency Virus', *Annals of International Medicine*, vol. 105, p. 969.

MONZON, OFELIA and CAPELLAN, JOSE M.B. (1987) 'Female-to-Female Transmission of HIV', *Lancet*, vol. 2, 4th July, pp. 40–1.

O'DONNELL, MARY, LEOFFLER, VAL., POLLOCK, KATER and SAUNDERS, ZIESEL (1980) *Lesbian Health Matters*, Santa Cruz, UP press.

O'SULLIVAN, SUE and PARMAR, PRATIBHA (1992) *Lesbians Talk (Safer) Sex*, London, Scarlet Press.

PATTON, CINDY (1985) Sex and Germs, Boston, South End Press.

PATTON, CINDY and KELLY, JANIS (1987) *Making It: A Woman's Guide to Sex in the Age of AIDS*, New York, The Crossing Press.

PERRY, SAMUEL, JACOBSBERG, LAWRENCE and FOGEL, KAREN (1989) 'Orogenital Transmission of Human Immunodeficiency Virus (HIV)' *Annals of International Medicine*, vol. 111, p. 951.

RICHARDSON, DIANE (1989) *Women and the AIDS Crisis*, 2nd ed., London, Pandora.

RICHARDSON, DIANE (1992) 'Constructing Lesbian Sexualities', in PLUMMER, KEN (Ed.) *Modern Homosexualities: Fragments of Lesbian and Gay Experience*, London, Routledge, pp. 187–99.

RICHARDSON, DIANE (1993) 'AIDS and Reproduction' in AGGLETON, PETER, DAVIES, PETER and HART, GRAHAM (Eds) *AIDS: Facing the Second Decade*, London, Falmer Press, pp. 99–108.

SABATINI, M.T., PATEL, K. and HIRSCHMAN, R. (1984) 'Kaposi's Sarcoma and T-Cell Lymphoma in an Immunodeficient Woman: A Case Report', *AIDS Research*, vol. 1, pp. 135-7.

SAGHIR, MARCEL T. and ROBINS, ELI (1973) *Male and Female Homosexuality: A Comprehensive Investigation*, Baltimore, Williams and Wilkins.

SASSE, H., IARDINO, R., CODICE, A., GHERARDI, C., FARCHI, F. and CHIAROTTI, F. (1992) 'Potential for Transmission of HIV Virus among Homo/Bisexual Women', paper given at the Second European Conference on Homosexuality and HIV: HIV Policy, Prevention, Care and Research: A Gay and Lesbian Perspective, Amsterdam, 14-16 February 1992.

SCHNEIDER, BETH (1992) 'Lesbian Politics and AIDS Work' in PLUMMER, KEN (Ed) *Modern Homosexualities: Fragments of Lesbian and Gay Experience*, London, Routledge, pp. 160–74.

SOLOMON, NANCY (1992) 'Risky Business: Should Lesbians Practise Safer Sex?', *Out/Look*, no. 15, Spring.

SPITZER, P.G. and WEINER, N.J. (1989) 'Transmission of HIV Infection from a Woman to a Man by Oral Sex', *New England Journal of Medicine*, vol. 320, p. 251.

STACEY, JACKIE (1991) 'Promoting Normality: Section 28 and the Regulation of Sexuality', in FRANKLIN, SARAH, LURY, CELIA and STACEY, JACKIE (Eds) *Off Centre: Feminism and Cultural Studies*, London, Hyman Unwin.

STERN, PHYLLIS NOERAGER (1993) 'Lesbian Health: What Are the Issues?', *Health Care for Women International*, vol. 14.

WELLINGS, KAYE, JOHNSON, ANNE, FIELD, J. and WANDSWORTH, J. (1994) *Sexual Behaivour in Britain*, Harmondsworth, Penguin.

Chapter 11

Against All Odds: HIV and Safer Sex Education for Women with Learning Difficulties

Michelle McCarthy

'Learning difficulties' is the preferred term for what used to be described in Britain as mental handicap. In an international context it can be used interchangeably with developmental disabilities, mental retardation (USA) and intellectual disability (Australia).

This chapter will first outline special concerns in relation to doing safer sex work with people with learning difficulties, as opposed to other groups in the population. The particular issues facing women will then be discussed. I will argue that a feminist understanding of the sexual lives of women with learning difficulties is critical to effective safer sex education. I argue that to undertake safer sex work with people with learning difficulties without a framework of sexual politics is easier, but misguided and ultimately unhelpful.

HIV and People with Learning Difficulties

There has been no research in Britain to ascertain the level of HIV infection amongst people with learning difficulties. Research in the USA (Kastner *et al.*, 1992) and anecdotal evidence in Britain suggests that the numbers of HIV-positive people with learning difficulties are very low. This offers no cause for complacency, however, and is a powerful argument *for* doing safer sex education, rather than against it. To wait until there are 'significant' numbers of people with learning difficulties infected with HIV before recognizing that this population had a need for safer sex education would be irresponsible in the extreme. Also, given that (as I shall argue later) HIV prevention cannot be done with people with learning difficulties in isolation from a more general exploration of sexual matters, it provides a much needed opportunity to offer people information about their bodies, their relationships, issues of abuse and consent, etc.

It is important to consider whether people with learning difficulties would need safer sex education aimed specially at them or whether they can make use of the information about HIV/AIDS and safer sex advice that is in general circulation. Obviously, people with learning difficulties are not a homogeneous group; there is great variation in levels of understanding and intellectual ability and therefore some people with learning difficulties may benefit from the general public information campaigns. Most, however, would not have gained from this. Having a learning difficulty, by definition, implies an impairment in learning, understanding, remembering and transferring knowledge and skills from one situation to another.

Generally speaking, safer sex education is most often thought of as giving people information so they can make their own choices and take responsibility for their own sexual behaviour. Many people with learning difficulties may not fully understand the information, however, or they may not remember it. In addition, they may be in a very poor position to exercise choice — because of a lack of comprehension, lack of skill and practice in making choices and/or because they lack any influence over their sexual partner(s). In recognition of these factors, there is a need for special initiatives with people with learning difficulties which will involve simplifying information, prioritizing safer sex messages and working on an individual basis.

The most obvious example of simplifying information occurs when trying to explain to people with learning difficulties what it is they are supposed to be protecting themselves and others from. Many people with learning difficulties do not know that sex between two people can have physiological consequences, e.g. pregnancy or sexually transmitted diseases. This lack of awareness may stem from never having received any sex education and also from the fact that the person's own experience, and that of their peer group, is probably that, in effect, there have never been any such consequences.

Many people with learning difficulties do not have clear concepts of disease, of time or of death. Telling them then that they could get an infection (HIV), which they will not be able to see or feel, but which, after some considerable period of time, may develop into a condition called AIDS which is life-threatening, is clearly not going to mean very much. In these circumstances, it is not necessary for people to be able to distinguish between HIV and AIDS. Accuracy may need to be sacrificed for the sake of getting the message across (Jacobs *et al.*, 1989). What matters most is that people learn how to protect themselves from something very serious. Consequently, HIV will usually not be mentioned at all, reference will only be made to AIDS, which many people with learning difficulties will already have heard of. I readily acknowledge that the confusion of terms HIV/AIDS and the equation 'AIDS = death' goes against the grain of general HIV education and if done without a good reason is certainly unsound practice. But the reality of the limited understanding of many people with learning difficulties must be accepted and worked with, not glossed over.

Giving information about oral sex is an example of the need to prioritize safer sex messages. HIV/AIDS educators in this country generally present oral sex as having a very low risk of transmission of HIV, but people are informed that a very small number of people are thought to have been infected in this way. People can therefore decide whether they want to use condoms or dental dams for protection and generally the vast majority of people do not.

The limited ability of people with learning difficulties to comprehend and weigh up these uncertainties, combined with the generally accepted very low risk of transmission of HIV, means that unprotected oral sex is presented as a safer sexual activity. Only unprotected vaginal and anal intercourse are prioritized as risks.

Individual safer sex education is very important for people with learning difficulties. My project's experience suggests strongly that watching a video, looking at a leaflet or posters (even those specifically aimed at this group) or talking about safer sex in a group are very unlikely to result in anybody with learning difficulties putting safer sex into practice. Individual sessions with a worker of the same sex over a period of several weeks or months have proved necessary to get to know the individual, their capabilities and limitations and their sexual practices. Areas of work will cover safer sex advice, including, but not limited to, information about condom use, practising (with a model penis) getting condoms on and off, making sure condoms are easily accessible thereafter, and, of utmost importance, negotiating safer sex.

Particular Issues for Women with Learning Difficulties

Three years' full-time experience of sex education work with women with learning difficulties has given me a very good picture of their sexual lives. My academic research and practical work have highlighted some very common features of the sexual experiences of women with learning difficulties. My own work is predominantly within long-stay hospitals, but discussions with colleagues working outside of institutions, and with women with learning difficulties themselves, confirm that these experiences are commonplace and not dependent on any one particular setting.

Women with learning difficulties rarely experience their sexuality in any positive way. Few seem to masturbate, and those who do so do not experience it as fulfilling. They usually believe it is wrong and dirty and that they will harm themselves by doing it. I have met no women with learning difficulties who have sex with other women, despite the fact that most of the women I meet live on women-only wards. This situation is not likely to be merely due to underreporting, as the women speak openly, and usually without prejudice, about men who have sex with men.

My academic research concerned sexual pleasure for women with learning difficulties and this is conspicuous by its absence. It is neither expected nor experienced by the overwhelming majority of the women with learning difficulties I have met. This is accepted by both the women themselves and their male partners as the norm. Related to this is the fact that none of the women or men with learning difficulties my project has met have been aware of the existence of the clitoris or of women's orgasms. American research confirms these findings (Andron, 1983; Timmers *et al.*, 1981).

Also apparent are extremely high levels of sexual abuse perpetrated against the women throughout their lives by fathers, brothers, male strangers and men with learning difficulties. The abuse, particularly by men with learning difficulties, with whom the women are often in close daily contact, is usually not perceived by the women as abusive, but rather as 'normal' sex.

The women with learning difficulties with whom I work most commonly have sex with men with learning difficulties, although it is not at all uncommon to find that some also have sex with men who do not have any kind of disability. These men either come into the hospital grounds with the express purpose of finding a sexual partner or they meet the women outside the grounds, sometimes in the local towns. Efforts are made by staff and the police to catch the men who come into the hospitals.

The process of events is that almost all heterosexual encounters, as described by both the women and the men with learning difficulties, are focused exclusively on the men's genitals. The women will rub the man's penis when or until he has an erection, penetration of an unlubricated vagina or anus follows and sex finishes with the man's orgasm. The whole sexual encounter is usually over within a few minutes, not least because people with learning difficulties are usually afforded no privacy and dignity for their sexual relations and so are obliged to snatch opportunities where they can. The lack of privacy is most apparent in large institutions, but is often just as much of a problem for people with learning difficulties living in community-based group homes or hostels or who live with their parents.

This is clearly a very depressing picture and I would argue that it is one that is only built up through working from a feminist perspective. The above, very detailed information on actual sexual experiences is rarely going to be *offered* by women or men with learning difficulties in the course of sex education. It is much more common simply to learn that people are having sex and the assumption is then often made that if people are doing it, they must like it, otherwise they would not do it. This assumption does seem to be true for the men but is rarely the case for the women themselves. The body of feminist knowledge built up over many years indicates that what is happening to women with learning difficulties now is not fundamentally different to what has happened for many other women across cultures and throughout history. Likewise, the body of feminist knowledge and skills that have been built up around the issue of sexual abuse (particularly the knowledge that the abuser is most often a known and trusted man and that abuse commonly takes place within the context of an existing, intimate relationship) has led me to ask women with learning difficulties what is actually going on for them.

Implications of Not Working from a Feminist Perspective

It is only by asking the right questions that you find out what sex is really like for women with learning difficulties. It is equally important to ask the same questions of the men they have sex with. It is not possible to talk to the men who do not have learning difficulties, as they are secretive in their behaviour and therefore not open to question. But as they are very clearly exploiting vulnerable women and are out to get their own sexual needs met, it does not seem unreasonable to conclude that they are not the most sensitive of sexual partners. The men with learning difficulties, however, when asked in detail about their sexual practices with women, give a clear picture that they are the ones who control the sexual activity, that it is for their pleasure and that the women's bodies, even those of their long-established girlfriends in some instances, are the tools to provide that pleasure. Few, if any, of the men our project has worked with know or care what women like sexually. This is not to paint a picture of men with learning difficulties as brutal monsters who deliberately set out to hurt women, but it is the case that during sex, the women's feelings, desires, pain or pleasure are irrelevant to them.

Without a framework of sexual politics and without an understanding of gender power relations, this kind of information is not gleaned. Consequently, I believe that much of the general sex education and specifically HIV education that is done with people with learning difficulties is not grounded in reality and is therefore not helpful.

For example, the most recent sex education resource by the person acknowledged to be the British expert in the field presents sex between men and women with learning difficulties as a loving act between two equals (Craft, 1991). It makes a passing reference that intercourse should not hurt anybody, but with an added note that if sufficient time is not allowed for 'foreplay' the women's vagina may get sore or hurt. In the section on condom use, it gives advice on how to teach people with learning difficulties how to use them, but offers nothing about the potential difficulties of negotiating safer sex. The suggestion is made that sex education can be easily done in mixed-sex groups and, throughout the pack, gender-neutral language is most commonly used; it is therefore implied that anybody can be abused by anybody else. Strictly speaking this may be true, but it masks the fact that the overwhelming majority of sexual abusers are male and that although men with learning difficulties are vulnerable to sexual abuse in a way that most adult men are not, it is *women* with learning difficulties who are most vulnerable to domination and abuse by their male peers, and not the other way around.

Within most heterosexual encounters it is the man who controls and directs what happens sexually and the woman who goes along with it, even though it may not be entirely what she wants or likes (Women's Action on AIDS Video, 1992). It takes a particularly confident and assertive woman to be able to tell a man what she wants sexually and it takes a particularly sensitive and respectful man to take any notice of her. To ignore the fact that this is just as likely to be the case for people with learning difficulties seems to me to be naive.

This situation is also a direct result of the traditional view of people with learning difficulties as asexual beings or eternal children. These ideas seem, thankfully, very dated now, and most concerned individuals and services strive to accord people with learning difficulties the adult status that is rightfully theirs. However, they are still often considered to be simply 'people' with learning difficulties, not women and men with different needs, interests and experiences. It is my contention that certainly with regard to their sexuality, women and men with learning difficulties have more in common with their non-disabled counterparts than they do with each other. Any sex education and HIV prevention work should reflect this.

What Does Feminist Safer Sex Education Look Like?

First and foremost, feminist safer sex education is offered by women to women. Despite Craft's confident assertion that 'no difficulty was reported' in her experience of mixed-sex education groups (Craft, 1991), this has not been my experience. Most of the groups I run for women with learning difficulties are fairly ambivalent at the start of the work about the potential inclusion of men in the group. However, once the group is under way and always at the end of the group's life, when asked if they would have preferred men in the group too, the answer is a loud and resounding 'NO'. The women feel that they would not have been able to talk so openly and honestly if men had been present and that they would have been embarrassed. The women from the London branch of People First (a self-advocacy organization for people with learning difficulties) state very clearly in their sexuality policies that they want women-only groups and more women staff, both for personal care and sex education (*People First Newsletter,* 1991).

Women's groups have a number of benefits and it is certainly possible for women to learn in groups what AIDS is about and the need for safer sex, but my experience suggests that if women are to be able to put what they have learned into practice, individual sessions are necessary. Working from a feminist perspective indicates that this work should also be along single-sex lines. Not only does this give the women with learning difficulties a greater chance of identifying with the safer sex advisor, it also offers an opportunity to look at shared life experiences — it can enable women with learning difficulties to see that some of their experiences, concerns and needs are more to do with them being a woman than to do with having a learning difficulty. This is by no means to imply that we are all the same and that women with learning difficulties do not live with particular constraints and disadvantages, but there are likely to be some points of commonality. It may also be the first time that a woman with learning difficulties gets to ask someone else about her sexual life. This model of sex education implies that the worker needs to be prepared to answer personal questions regarding her own sexuality. Whilst issues of confidentiality and personal embarrassment need to be taken into consideration, it is hardly fair or likely to foster an atmosphere of openness and trust if the flow of personal revelations are all one-way. A feminist approach to this work means not seeing other women merely as clients, subjects of research or people to be passively helped.

Working along single-sex lines has the added advantage of making male workers responsible for dealing with men's sexuality.

Moving on from style to content, it is important that HIV prevention is not done in isolation from a more general discussion of sex and relationships. (I have neither met nor heard of any people with learning difficulties who inject drugs, so my own work, and all the specialist HIV education resources, concentrates solely on sexual transmission of the virus.)

Detailed HIV preventive work which is aimed towards achieving a change in sexual behaviour is best done with people with learning difficulties when they are already sexually active or when it seems they are likely to be having sex in the very near future. Whilst this might be considered as having left things a bit late, it has to be weighed against the risk of educating people 'too early'. If people with learning difficulties are given information about HIV and safer sex at a time when they are not sexually active, it will be harder for them to understand as they may have no concrete experiences to relate the abstract information to. Moreover, they may have forgotten it by the time an opportunity arises to put it into practice.

In order to maximize the possibility of giving effective safer sex advice, it is essential to get as comprehensive a picture as possible of the woman's sexual life. This involves asking what kind of sex she has and with whom — the latter point does not mean you need to know the names of the partners, but it is important to know, for example, whether it is an individual man from her peer group or a stranger who picks her up when she leaves her day centre since this will make a difference to the rest of the work.

It will also be important to know if she is having sex with one man in the context of an established relationship or with more than one, where the contact is purely or primarily sexual. Women should not be questioned like this for the sake of it, or to satisfy the worker's curiosity, but because it is important to know the context of her sexual activity when trying to enable her to negotiate and protect herself.

There is a need to explore which sexual activities she likes and dislikes. Particular attention needs to be paid to any sexual activity which she engages in without liking/wanting it. The most common example of this, in my experience, is anal intercourse. There is a need to look at why this happens and what stops her from saying no to an experience that may be physically painful and/or emotionally distressing. Commonly, as for many other women, the reasons are that women with learning difficulties fear verbal and/or physical abuse and/or the loss of the relationship.

I have had discussions with HIV workers (sadly women as well as men) who see their role as purely the prevention of HIV, excluding involvement with wider aspects of people's sexual lives. I believe this is not compatible with working from a feminist perspective and can be seen as collusion with any abuse, exploitation or deception that may be taking place. When a woman reveals that she is having sex which she neither wants nor enjoys, the focus of the work should be on helping her find ways to make that stop, not on ways to make it safer in terms of HIV.

If it is ascertained that a women does like the sex she is having or is going to continue with it anyway (because, even with support, facing the consequences of not doing so are too difficult), then the work on safer sex begins.

At the beginning of this chapter, I outlined some important points with regard to simplifying and prioritizing information. Only vaginal and anal intercourse are presented as risky activities; everything else is described as safe. The problem is that often there is not anything else. As I explained earlier, lack of private space and time means that sexual encounters are often hurried and the fact that the men control what happens during this limited time means that they get what they want, or perhaps the only thing they know, which is almost always penetrative sex. Whilst it remains very important to talk about non-penetrative sex, safer sex advisors need to be realistic and acknowledge that the sensual/sexual exploration of your own and your partner's body is just not feasible in certain circumstances.

At this point, it is important to make a comment about women with learning difficulties and oral sex. None of the women with learning difficulties I have met have ever experienced a man's mouth on their genitals. Many women with learning difficulties have experienced a man's penis in their mouths and this is an act which they unanimously loathe. Every woman has said she finds it disgusting and horrible and, very significantly, most of the women say they refuse to do it and the men my project works with confirm this picture. Quite where or why the women find the strength to refuse this particular sexual act, when they tolerate others they dislike, I do not know. But, in my work, I am always very encouraging if women make this stand and I try to help them build on it to assert themselves in other areas. However, in terms of promoting safer sex, unless the women are able to persuade the men to give them oral sex (and in view of everything else that happens this seems highly unlikely), then this particular non-penetrative alternative is pretty much out of the picture.

As vaginal and anal intercourse are likely to be the main components of a lot of people's sexual activity, condom use clearly plays an important part in any safer sex advice. With people with learning difficulties, practical teaching methods are usually most successful, using a model penis so that they can practise getting them on and off. Many people with learning difficulties find this very difficult to do and, in fact, even after much teaching and practice, cannot do it. Nonetheless, most women with learning difficulties I have worked with have felt comfortable with the idea of knowing how to put a condom on a man and have been keen to learn.

If women do learn how to use condoms, the safer sex advisor needs to consider how condoms can be made accessible to the woman, as and when she needs them. Unlike many others, people with learning difficulties do not always have the opportunity, financial resources or skills to go to shops and buy them. The worker needs to give thought as to how the woman can be perhaps supported to go to a Family Planning Clinic, or how a residential or day service might make condoms available free or at a subsidized cost. There are a number of options, few of which are without their difficulties, but at the end of the day, there is no point in teaching people how and why they should use condoms if they do not have easy access to them.

Teaching women with learning difficulties the practicalities of safer sex is only the first step in the process of effective safer sex education. They need to understand, and in my experience are only too well aware, that even if *they* want to have safer sex, the man may not want to or see the need to and so some kind of negotiation will be necessary. Negotiating safer sex with men is something even very articulate women often find difficult. For a woman with learning difficulties who may not have good communication skills, particularly if she is trying to negotiate with a man with learning difficulties who may have limited understanding and poor communication skills himself, things are a lot more difficult.

Again, a practically based approach is likely to be most effective. Using pictures of different kinds of sexual activities, role play involving the woman herself, or watching a video of role plays (see for example, Young Adult Institute Video, 1987) can give the woman an opportunity to practise how she might suggest condom use, how she might explain why this is important and how she might proceed if there is initial or prolonged resistance from her partner.

Women with learning difficulties need to be helped to look at their own particular situation realistically and to consider to what extent they can request or insist upon safer sex and to consider what their options are either if they are unable to express their wishes and/or if the man does not comply with them. The reality may be that their options are few and not particularly positive in their outcome, but the reality has to be faced.

From the title of this chapter and all that has been said, it should be clear that doing HIV prevention work with women with learning difficulties is no easy task. The odds really are stacked against a successful outcome and this is reflected in my project's work, which, despite ample time, resources and committed workers, cannot say with any confidence that many, if indeed any, women with learning difficulties are regularly practising safer sex. However, despite what seems a very depressing picture, it is still vitally important that women with learning difficulties get a chance to speak about their sexual lives, the positive and negative things that they experience. They need the opportunity to talk with other women and learn that they do not simply have to service men's sexual needs and that sex should be a positive, dignified and safe activity for them too. Until women with learning difficulties have taken these messages on board, and it may take months or even years, they are in a very poor position to even start thinking about protecting themselves from HIV. Safer sex education for people with learning difficulties which does not explicitly acknowledge and try to challenge the power of men in most heterosexual relationships is doing a disservice to women with learning difficulties. A feminist perspective and a commitment to equal opportunities offer some hope for progress and change.

References

ANDRON, L. (1983) 'Sexuality Counselling with Developmentally Disabled Couples', in CRAFT, A. and CRAFT, M. (Eds) *Sex Education and Counselling for Mentally Handicapped People,* Tunbridge Wells, Costello.

CRAFT, A. and Nottingham SLD Sex Education Project (1991) *Living Your Life — A Sex Education and Personal Development Programme for Students with Severe Learning Difficulties,* Cambridge, Development Aids Learning.

JACOBS, R., SAMOWITZ, P., LEVY, J.M. and LEVY, P.H. (1989) 'Developing an AIDS Prevention Education Program for Persons with Developmental Disabilities', *Mental Retardation,* vol. 27, no. 4, pp. 233-7.

KASTNER, T., NATHANSON, R.S. and MARCHETTI, A.G. (1992) 'Epidemiology of HIV Infection in Adults with Developmental Disabilities', in CROCKER, A.C., COHEN, H.J. and KASTNER, T.A. *HIV Infection and Developmental Disabilities: A Resource for Service Providers,* Baltimore, Paul Brookes Publishers.

PEOPLE FIRST NEWSLETTER (London) (1991) Winter.

TIMMERS, R. *et al.,* (1981) 'Sexual Knowledge and Behaviours of Developmentally Disabled Adults Living in a Normalised Apartment Setting', *Sexuality and Disability,* vol. 4, no. 1.

Michelle McCarthy

Videos

WOMEN'S ACTION ON AIDS, (1992) Mouthing Off (35 minutes). Produced by the Leeds AIDS Advice. Distributed by Concord Video.

YOUNG ADULT INSTITUTE (1987) *Teaching People with Disabilities to Better Protect Themselves,* New York.

Chapter 12

Time for a Makeover?
Women and Drugs in the Context of AIDS

Sheila Henderson

This chapter examines the subject of women's illicit drug use in the context of HIV/AIDS. There are many aspects of this topic which still need to be addressed, including the stigma which still surrounds illegal drug use, the inadequacy of service provision, the effects of drug use on pregnancy and a range of other women's health matters, the lack of knowledge about the relationship between street drugs and a compromised immune system — and between these two factors and maintenance drugs such as methadone (a heroin substitute), AZT and other treatments. However, my aim in this chapter is to spark off discussion and debate concerning a wider feminist agenda on drugs use and HIV/AIDS. This will be done by considering the broader impact of both feminism and AIDS on the development and context of services and policies relating to women drug users, and by asking how appropriate these are for the 1990s.

Pictures of Women and Drugs Before AIDS

Before considering the impact of AIDS, it is important to establish, however briefly, the historical context of women's illicit drug use. What were the images and moral tone surrounding women's drug use before the intervention of HIV? How was it conceptualized and constructed by social policy?

The history of women's involvement in illicit drug use is fascinating, although poorly documented (Kohn, 1992; Palmer and Horowitz, 1982). Popular media images of women and illicit drugs have tended to involve two main themes: the tragic victim, passive in her drug use, and the more active, hence morally culpable and sexualized, 'bad girl'. Alternative or counter-cultural media, on the other hand, have been more likely to glamorize active drug use, emphasizing the tragic heroines of popular music such as Billie Holliday, Nico and Janis Joplin, seemingly bent on self-destruction.

It is still the case that, compared to women, men can use a wider range of drugs in a wider range of social settings with less social reprimand. The association of women with drugs can lead to another association — that of sexual deviancy. This in turn can generate added condemnation, not only from society in general but also from male peers, especially in some injecting scenes. Street drugs have always tended to score high on the moral disapproval scale (with heroin scoring highest) while other drugs, such as alcohol, tobacco, tranquillizers, anti-depressants and slimming pills, have tended to line up on the scale according to historical twists and fashions. Smoking, for example, especially during pregnancy, is now widely viewed as morally reprehensible behaviour, yet as recently as the 1970s it was considered to be perfectly respectable.

Prior to the involvement of the women's health movement in the drugs field, women were not much in evidence in British drugs services, policies and literature. Early studies of consumers of services put the proportion of women to men at approximately one in four (Blumberg, 1981) or later at one in three (Glantz and Taylor, 1986; Sheehan *et al.*, 1988). In general, women were of concern only if they were pregnant or involved in prostitution. The literature, dominated by medical and psychological perspectives, explained women's drug use as a 'deviation' from 'normal' femininity due to mental or physical deficiencies or disease (Rosenbaum, 1981; Cuskey, 1982). Service provision based on these perspectives tended to be preoccupied with the effects of drug use on pregnancy outcomes, with priority given to the health of the baby (Blenheim Project, 1988, p. 1). Such a response was still evident in HIV-positive women's personal accounts of experiences of pregnancy in the early day of the HIV/AIDS epidemic.

The Impact of the Women's Health Movement

Writings coming from the women's health movement have been an important resource for women organizing around HIV/AIDS. They were also an important resource for women involved in the area of alcohol and illicit drugs in the 1970s. The starting point for these women's critique of drugs policies was the now familiar assertion that studies of drugs use ignored gender as a significant factor and extrapolated from the male experience. A key article claimed that 'the extent, context and experience of female drug use remain invisible' (Perry, 1979, p. 4) and equated women's drug dependence with broader social forms of dependency:

> Drug dependent females are seen as characteristically pathetic, passive, psychologically and socially inadequate, isolated and incapable of shouldering responsibilities . . . These images are drawn from a view of women's major role as centrally responsible for the 'private' side of life — housework, childcare, emotional support and family servicing . . . the illegal addict is seen as first rejecting and then being rendered incapable of performing these functions effectively which is initially wilfully perverse and then inescapably pathetic. . . . Female dependence is a reality — female drug dependence is an inappropriate and undesirable side-effect to be redirected to more convenient and controllable forms of dependence. (Perry, 1979, p. 1)

Sociological research on women's drug use has not developed significantly in the fourteen years since Perry's article. A study published in 1981 (Rosenbaum, 1981) was until recently (Taylor, 1993) the most notable in-depth sociological study of how injecting drug use fits into women's lives.

The history of the impact of the women's health movement on the provision of drug services is largely ancedotal. However, it suggests that a range of initiatives were developed around the country in the 1980s to meet the needs of women drug users. Women's networking around the issue culminated in the establishment of Drugs, Alcohol, Women, Nationally (DAWN) in 1979. DAWN provided an information and advice service until the end of 1990, when it ceased to exist as an organization. At the time of writing, there are plans to revive it in the shape of a national network. The DAWN survey of facilities for women using drugs in London (DAWN, 1984) found that, of 254 agencies, 154 had no service actively targeting women.

The impact was also felt at the official level. The Advisory Council on the Misuse of Drugs Report in 1984 drew attention to the invisibility of gender issues:

> We are also concerned with other groups at risk of misusing drugs. In the 1960s and 1970s drug misuse among women was not considered an area of particular interest. Researchers and

policy makers have often assumed that hypotheses and policies drawn up in response to male drug misuse are equally applicable to women . . . the women's movement has drawn attention to the need to conceptualise 'social problems' (such as the drug problem) from the point of view of women's interest and position in society . . . we consider that this literature raises important issues not adequately dealt with in earlier male-centred work. (p. 23)

However, this official recognition was not accompanied by any significant increase in initiatives addressing women's drug use. It has taken the advent of HIV/AIDS to accomplish this.

Responses to Women and Drugs in the Light of AIDS

In order to understand the impact of AIDS on women drug users, we have to consider its impact on the drugs field in general. England is one of the few contries where harm reduction — as a concept and a set of practical measures — has in recent years been a pragmatic policy response to illicit drug use. The impetus for this came specifically from official and popular concern to limit the spread of HIV and AIDS in injecting drug users to the wider population. Thus the (partial) official acceptance of safer and/or controlled drug use as an appropriate treatment goal was fuelled by a public health agenda. This top-down strategy differed markedly from the grass-roots mobilization of gay communities.

The response of drug services to HIV/AIDS has been described elsewhere (Donoghoe *et al.*, 1992; Ettorre, 1990; Macgregor *et al.*, 1991; O'Hare *et al.*, 1992; Stimson, 1990). In summary, key developments involved an emphasis upon 'user-friendliness', multi-agency work and making contact with drug users through the use of outreach and detached work, needle and syringe exchanges and the 'flexible prescribing' of maintenance drugs such as methadone (a heroin substitute). A shift towards community-based services begun by the Central Funding Initiative — a government funding initiative from 1986 to 1989 responsible for a major growth in drug services (Macgregor *et al.*, 1991) was also consolidated.

What consequences have these developments had for women drug users? More generally, it would appear from informal feedback from women working in the field that these funding-led developments have refocused attention on injecting drug use to the detriment of much previous work around tranquillizers and the use of amphetamines or amphetamine-like drugs for the purposes of slimming.

Meanwhile the more specific impact on women who inject drugs is difficult to gauge given the absence of national studies or published overviews. A report on the Central Funding Initiative (CFI) (Macgregor *et al.*, 1991) presents attendance statistics for the new CFI drug agencies for the period 1986-9. The overall male to female ratio was 1.6 to 1 among clients but this varied between types of service. Residential rehabilitation houses had the poorest ratio (4m:1f) whilst drop-in advice and counselling (or 'street') agencies performed best at 1.3m:1f. However, these were very early figures. Current statistics are collated by the Regional Drug Misuse Databases but there are problems of under-reporting and national summary tables have not been published at the time of writing. The North West Regional Drug Misuse Database reveals a widening of the gender gap from 1990 to 1992. The male:female ratio for attenders was 2.6:1 in 1990, but 3.2:1 in 1992. This could be due to a fall in the number of women using drugs in the North-West or, more likely given current trends, a decline in the services attractive to women. The Regional Databases also hold information on the gender of people attending for maintenance prescriptions but, again, these are not currently available as published national reviews.

Evaluation of the other main plank of the harm reduction strategy, the government's three-year pilot of syringe exchange schemes in England, gives little indication that this service increased contact with women. Despite the fact that this 'shopping' role could well have been expected to fall to women given traditional female roles, the attendance figures give a male:female ratio of 4:1 (Donoghoe *et al.*, 1992).

In 1989, service providers were given an official spur to make their service more woman-friendly. The second of two reports by the Advisory Council on the Misuse of Drugs, *AIDS and Drug Misuse* (Advisory Council on the Misuse of Drugs, 1989) recommended that 'Drug services should review their policies to ensure they are receptive to the needs of women' (p. 41). The report highlighted reasons why services are less accessible to women:

because they find the service off-putting and not understanding of their needs; because it is difficult to find somebody to look after their children; or because they are frightened that their children will be taken into care if they admit to having a drug problem. Evidence indicates that women are far more likely to attend services which consciously aim to attract them; unfortunately many services inadvertently deter them. (pp. 23–4)

Recommendations were made for improving access, such as women-only sessions, availability of women doctors and counsellors, provision of creche facilities, family planning advice and well-informed counselling for pregnant HIV-positive women. The DAWN survey awaiting publication will perhaps give us some inkling of the initial impact of these recommendations.

More possible to ascertain are the *forms* of service provision which have developed following HIV/AIDS funding. In particular, new out-of-agency working methods, variously described as outreach or detached work, have proliferated. Such initiatives have focused on working with prostitute women on the streets, but also in massage parlours and saunas, even providing special drop-ins (Plant, 1990; McIver, 1992). Such projects have enabled prostitutes to access primary health care, free condoms, syringe exchange, various drug treatment options and a range of informal support.

The historically macho nature of much 'street work' has also been criticized as an inappropriate means of contacting women drug users more generally. Methods developed in other fields, notably in the context of homelessness, have emerged:

> When I was a detached . . . worker I spent a lot of time in shops, cafes, community centres, launderettes, various agencies and in people's houses. Saying that you've spent all afternoon in the launderette isn't half as impressive as saying you've been out all night 'on the streets', but it tends to be where the women are . . . (Yates and Gilman, 1990, p. 20)

Some Drug Dependency Units (DDUs) and Community Drug Teams (CDTs), best known for their role in dispensing prescriptions for maintenance drugs, have also made special efforts to contact women. These have tended to emphasize the needs of pregnant women and prostitute women and have included liaison with other specialist drug and generic agencies such as local maternity and gynaecological services; flexible and prioritized appointment systems; non-medical referrals; home visits from staff; and support with stabilizing drug use. In one case at least, a specialist worker supports women who wish to come off drugs and leave prostitution by providing practical assistance with housing difficulties, employment alternatives, keeping hospital appointments, etc. (Ruben, 1990).

Pregnant drug users have historically evoked the spectre of the 'unfit mother'. With the advent of HIV/AIDS, this reaction has been amplified. The early, now disproven, medical information which suggested that women with the virus would almost certainly go on to develop AIDS in pregnancy and infect their child did much to exacerbate the situation. HIV-positive women who injected or had injected, and became pregnant were generally condemned and steered towards termination without the option of informed and supported choice. The situation has recently improved, spearheaded in particular by a model of care developed in Glasgow. An obstetric service was transformed into a community-based women's reproductive health service, offering support with housing, employment, financial and legal problems, as well as other health needs, on site (Hepburn, 1990). Within this framework, it has been possible to challenge the standard view that coming off drugs during the first or third trimester of pregnancy will damage the baby. Pregnancy outcomes have been the same or better among women who have taken the option of coming off drugs (Hepburn, 1993) but, most importantly, women have been in a position to make informed choices.

The above is not intended as a comprehensive summary of all initiatives for women drug users since AIDS became an issue. Some specialist residential services have attempted to provide better facilities for women, as have some voluntary AIDS agencies. There has been some improvement in service provision; however, there is still ample room for future development in many directions.

Reaching an Impasse

Clearly feminism has had an impact on the ethos and provision of services for women in the context of drug use and HIV/AIDS. The advent of HIV/AIDS focused attention on women's drug use but, in so doing, largely restricted the scope of that focus to injecting drug use. Feminism has had a broad impact on drug use and drug services. Sketching future directions requires a closer look at the kind of feminism underlying these developments. How has it been expressed and how has it changed over the last twenty years?

Referring back to the first official reference to the need to focus on women's drug use (Advisory Council on the Misuse of Drugs, 1984) highlights an important area of change: 'The potential contribution to drug prevention of women's consciousness-raising and self-help within the context of the women's movement, and the possibility that women's organisations may act as an alternative to problematic drug use, are areas deserving closer study' (Advisory Council on the Misuse of Drugs, 1984, p. 24).

The suggestion that the women's movement, in true emancipatory style, could serve as a form of drug prevention (a 'go to a womb workshop and throw away your works' approach!) no longer receives public airing. However, two of the most recent books on women and drug use (Ettorre, 1993; Sargent, 1992) suggest that other perspectives have not changed (although they have been absorbed more deeply into academia). The concept of dependence remains central and the entirely negative outlook arising from this has become entrenched. This process of entrenchment has been aided by many factors, significant among them the greater currency of sociological perspectives which view drug use as a compensation for social deficit such as unemployment or lack of housing (Mugford and O'Malley, 1990). Within such a conceptual framework, the possibility of positive reasons for women's drug use tend to slip from view.

In an attempt to set a feminist agenda on women and drug use, Ettorre (1989), considered the 'need to look perhaps more closely at the pleasurable effects of substances and in particular to ask ourselves why and how women experience their substance use as pleasurable' (p. 598). However, her conclusion that 'pleasure for most women appears as a subverted or hidden reality' (p. 599), together with her initial premise that 'there are few public settings, contexts or mechanisms whereby women can address their experiences in terms of the choices they make or the benefits they receive from their consumption of substances' (p. 598) leave the more optimistic reader high and dry on the pleasure front once again.

It may seem out of place to speak about pleasure in the context of drug use and/or HIV but pleasure is nonetheless an important ingredient. It is not only implicated in the relationship between sex and drugs but also in the context of relationships in general and the minutae of everyday life. Feminist analysis has been good at *deconstructing* pleasure but not so good at *re*construction. Feminist perspectives on drug use have ignored positive elements such as pleasure, fun and the active choices women make and in so doing have been limited in their scope. This in turn has had consequences for service provision.

Consulting the Consumers

A colleague of mine finally achieved a longstanding ambition in 1992 when she organized a women-only programme for her service. She thought this necessary for reasons which are now familiar. She knew there were many potential female clients but they were not using the service in any significant numbers. Seven young women aged between 17 and 24 years eventually attended the three-week programme. All received pre- and post-programme counselling. Most were heroin injectors and involved with the criminal justice system. At one point, my colleague sought their views on what they as women wanted out of drug services. Their replies included the usual 'choice of a male or female drug worker' and 'local clinics/home visits and evening sessions' but also 'not being identified by my hormones' and 'not so bloody laid back — tighter controls and expectations'. The group also had a clear view of women drug workers: 'vegetarian, socialist, feminist, wear glasses, dress scruffily, are middle-class, not touched by money problems and animal rights/ environment activists'. Feminists, in their opinion, were 'butch, veggy, all have dogs/are animal friendly, live in scruffy accommodation, wear DM's and glasses, buy the *Guardian* , are skinheads and mindbenders who corrupt 'nice' women and hate men — lesbians'!

This is hardly a representative sample of women who use drug services but these comments do touch a nerve which goes far beyond the drugs field. Recent surveys (Beloff *et al.*, 1993) and articles in women's magazines have shown that while feminist *ideas* are popular today, *feminists* get a bad press. This negative image of feminists has currency and is often used to describe what they are *not*. If we are concerned with setting a feminist agenda in the HIV/AIDS context, we have to take this very real turn of events seriously. The dour 'womb workshop' approach to women's health lacks popular appeal and could well be an important factor in women's low take-up of drug services, including many women-only initiatives. Meanwhile, feminist attempts to take the moral judgment out of women's drug use and HIV-related matters have often involved an alternative form of moral policing; laying down rules for what is appropriate female as well as male behaviour. It could be time to admit that we have been high on rhetoric and dogma but low on practical engagement with the everyday lives of many women and men, in particular those of younger generations.

Drug Use and Tomorrow's Generations

There has been a major boom in youth drugtaking in recent years and young women figure as much as young men. Young women are increasingly more likely to be smokers than are their male peers and are as likely to drink alcohol. They are also as likely to have tried an illegal drug — in some cases, more likely (Measham *et al.*, 1993). My own research over the last one and a half years (e.g. Henderson, 1993) has put me in touch with young women (and men) of 15 to 25 years old, from a range of social backgrounds. These young people have accessed feminist ideas via many sources — magazines and other popular media, books, peers, education and parents. They do not think of these ideas as being feminist but as simply commonsense. While the present economic climate may have reduced their economic opportunities and sexual equality has not generally been achieved, these young women have higher expectations than much feminist analysis would ascribe to them. Compared to older generations, many young women today take their comparative independence and confidence for granted.

Within the 'dance drugs' culture, the young women I interviewed varied in the frequency, quantity, range and duration of their drug use. Most had used Ecstasy, amphetamine and LSD on a weekly basis for periods ranging from three months to three years. The majority smoked tobacco and cannabis on a regular basis and had little taste for alcohol. These young women's participation in the 'scene' was more equal with that of men than previous accounts of drug use and youth culture would lead us to expect. They were generally present in greater numbers and were as likely to have been introduced to the culture and the drugs by female as by male friends. Young women in the 'scene' come from a range of class, race and ethnic backgrounds; they participate in low-level dealing; they are more likely to access the scene via a crowd of friends of mixed or single gender than simply via a boyfriend. Drug use for them is one part of a popular culture which involves music, clothes, magazines etc. and is sustained by large sections of the high street retail and leisure industries etc. This contrasts sharply with current perspectives on drug use in which women play bit parts as victims and men star as socially marginal but sometimes admirable rogues. It also raises important questions about current feminist approaches. Clearly this is a specific culture of drug use with its own dynamics. However, understanding it can help to reevaluate feminist perspectives on drug use in the light of AIDS and, perhaps more importantly, develop more appropriate services.

Accentuating the Positive: Moving Forward

Personal testimonies from women with the virus have made many contributions but one is particularly pertinent to this discussion — the necessity to emphasize the positive and retain a sense of humour. It is possible to apply this positive perspective to the general issue of women's drug use and build on it by drawing on lessons from the 'dance drug' culture. First, we need to put pleasure firmly back into the drug use equation. For many young women, drug use is part of recreation. What is more, this is recreation in which they can operate with more than a modicum of power. However, pleasure and drug use are sometimes accompanied by sex and risk. So the second task is to examine the interrelationship between drugs and sex and risk, but from a perspective which recognizes different cultures and types of drug use. Drug use is not synonymous with injecting. Third, the apparent increase in sexual equality in the 'dance drug' culture serves as an important reminder that dependence is not the inevitable lot of women. Making false assumptions of dependency can lead to an undesirable paternalistic or patronizing response from service providers. Fourth, understanding the increased range of options open to young women in this youth culture necessarily involves consideration of how young men have changed. Finally, understanding this mainstream youth culture is vital for its holds a key to future drugtaking patterns and requirements from drug services.

This chapter has introduced pointers for giving feminist perspectives on drug use a much-needed 'make-over' and bringing them into line with the realities of modern life. Asking about fun and pleasure, about shifts and changes in relations between the sexes, about the detail of men's behaviour and experience, and about the variation in gender dynamics in different drug using contexts poses a constructive challenge. These questions need to be addressed in existing policy and service provision. Effective HIV/AIDS prevention strategies could depend on it.

References

ADVISORY COUNCIL ON THE MISUSE OF DRUGS (1984) *Prevention*, London, HMSO.

ADVISORY COUNCIL ON THE MISUSE OF DRUGS (1989) *AIDS and Drug Misuse: Part Two*, London, HMSO.

BELOFF, H., CLARK, A., MACDONALD, M. and SIANN, G. (1993) *Convergences and Divergences: Gender Differences in Perceptions of Feminism*, Paper given to the British Psychological Society Annual Conference, April.

BLENHEIM PROJECT (1988) *Changing Gear: A Book for Women Who Use Drugs Illegally*, London, Blenheim Project.

BLUMBERG, H. (1981) 'The Characterisation of People Coming to Treatment', in EDWARDS, G. and BUSCH, C. (Eds) *Drug Problems in Britain: A Review of Ten Years*, London, Academic Press.

BROOM, D. and STEVENS, A. (1991) 'Doubly Deviant', *The International Journal on Drug Policy*, vol. 2, no. 4, (Jan-Feb), pp. 25-7.

BURY, J., MORRISON, V. and MCLACHLAN, S. (1992) *Working with Women and AIDS*, London, Routledge.

CUSKEY, W. (1982) 'Female Addiction: A Review of the Literature', *Journal of Addictions and Health*, vol. 3, no. 1, pp. 3-33.

DAWN (1984) *Survey of Facilities for Women Using Drugs (Including Alcohol) in London*, London, DAWN.

DONOGHOE, M., DOLAN, K. and STIMSON, G. (1992) *The Impact of Syringe Exchange Schemes in England: Service Delivery and Organisation, Client Characteristics and HIV Risk Behaviour*, report to the Department of Health, London, Centre for Research on Drugs and Health Behaviour.

ETTORRE, B. (1989) 'Women and Substance Use/Abuse: Towards a Feminist Perspective or How to Make Dust Fly', *Women's Studies International Forum*, vol. 12, no. 6, pp. 593–602.

ETTORRE, B. (1990) *Service Development for AIDS and Drugs*, paper presented to one-day seminar on AIDS and Drugs at Centre for Extra-Mural Studies, Birkbeck College, London.

ETTORRE, B. (1993) *Women and Substance Abuse*, Basingstoke, Macmillan.

GLANZ, A. and TAYLOR, C. (1986) 'Findings of a National Survey of the Role of General Practitioners in the Treatment of Opiate Misuse: Extent of Contact with Opiate Misusers', *British Medical Journal*, 293, pp. 427–30.

HAIN, S., LOTT, P. and MARSDEN, R. (1992) 'It Came from Outer Space!': Perspectives from the General Population and Generic Health and Welfare Professionals in England, in DORN, N., HENDERSON, S. and SOUTH, N. (Eds) *AIDS: Women, Drugs and Social Care*, London, Falmer Press.

HENDERSON, S. (1993) 'Luvdup and Deelited: Responses to Drug Use in the Second Decade', in AGGLETON, P., DAVIES, P. and HART, G. (Eds) *AIDS: The Second Decade*, London, Falmer Press.

HEPBURN, M. (1990) 'Obstetrics Drug Use and HIV', in HENDERSON, S. (Ed.) *Women, HIV, Drugs: Practical Issues*, London, ISDD, pp. 45–51.

HEPBURN, M. (1993) *Management of Drug Use in Pregnancy*, poster presentation P70, First International Meeting on Practical Obstetrics, Paris, May.

KOHN, M. (1992) *Dope Girls: The Birth of the British Drug Underground*, London, Lawrence and Wishart.

MACGREGOR, S., ETTORRE, B., COOMBER, R., CROSIER, A. and LODGE, H. (1991) *Drug Services in England and the Impact of the Central Funding Initiative*, London, ISDD.

MCIVER, N. (1992) 'Developing a Service for Prostitutes in Glasgow', in BURY, J., MORRISON, V. and MCLACHLAN, S. (Eds) *Working with Women and AIDS*, London, Routledge.

MEASHAM, F., NEWCOMBE, R. and PARKER, H. (1993) 'The post-heroin generation', *Druglink*, 8(3), pp. 16–17.

MUGFORD, S. and O'MALLEY, P. (1990) 'Policies Unfit for Heroin?', *International Journal on Drug Policy*, vol. 2, no. 1, pp. 16–22.

NEWCOMBE, R., MEASHAM, F. and PARKER, H. (1992) 'Preliminary Findings of the First Stage of a Longitudinal Survey of 776 14-15 year olds in the North West of England in 1991', paper given to the British Sociological Association Health in Europe Conference, University of Edinburgh, September.

O'HARE, P., NEWCOMBE, R., MATTHEWS, A., BUNING, E. and DRUCKER, E. (Eds) (1992) *The Reduction of Drug-Related Harm*, London, Routledge.

OPPENHEIMER, E. (1991) 'Alcohol and Drug Misuse among Women — An Overview', *British Journal of Psychiatry*, vol. 158, no. 10, pp. 36–44.

O'SULLIVAN, S. and THOMSON, K. (Eds) (1992) *Positively Women: Living with AIDS*, London, Sheba.

PALMER, C. and HOROWITZ, M. (1982) *Shaman Woman, Mainline Lady*, New York, Quill.

PERRY, L. (1979) *Women and Drug Use: An Unfeminine Dependency*, London, ISDD.

PLANT, M. (Ed.) (1990) *AIDS, Drugs and Prostitution*, London, Routledge.

RUBEN, S. (1990) 'Drug Dependency Units' in HENDERSON, S. (Ed.) *Women, HIV, Drugs: Practical Issues*, London, ISDD, pp. 52–7.

RIEDER, I. and RUPPELT, P. (Eds) (1989) *Matters of Life and Death*, London, Virago.

ROSENBAUM, M. (1981) *Women on Heroin*, New Brunswick, Rutgers University Press.

RYAN, L. (1991) *Desperately Seeking Services? A Directory of HIV Services for Women in the Thames Regions*, The Women's HIV/AIDS Network, London, Health Education Authority.

SARGENT, M. (1992) *Women, Drugs and Policy in Sydney, London and Amsterdam,* Aldershot, Avebury.

SHEEHAN, M., OPPENHEIMER, E. and TAYLOR, C. (1988) 'Who Comes for Treatment: Drug Misusers at Three London Clinics', *British Journal of Addiction,* vol. 83, pp. 311–20.

STIMSON, G. (1990) 'AIDS and HIV: The Challenge for British Drug Services', *British Journal of Addiction,* vol. 83, no. 3, pp. 329–51.

SUNDAY MIRROR (1989) *The AIDS Timebomb. Courts Let this Girl Go Free To Go Back On Game,* 13 August, p. 9.

TAYLOR, A. (1993) *Women Drug Users,* Oxford, Clarendon Press.

THE STAR (1986) *Children of the Damned,* 1 May, p. 1.

WOMEN AND HIV/AIDS NETWORK (1990) *Proceedings of the Second National Conference.*

YATES, R. and GILMAN, M. (1990) *Seeing More Drug Users: Outreach Work and Beyond,* London, ISDD.

Some Useful Organizations in Britain

Body Positive
51b Philbeach Gardens
London SW5 9EB
Tel: 071 835 1045 (office)
      071 373 9124 (helpline daily 7 p.m. to 10 p.m.)

Body Positive is a self-help organization providing information and support to men, women and children affected by HIV and AIDS. There is a Body Positive Women's Group which meets regularly for mutual support. Creche facilities and transport can be provided.

George House Trust
P.O. Box 201
Manchester M60 1PU
Tel: 061 839 4340 (office)
      061 839 2442 (helpline Mon-Fri 7 p.m. to 10 p.m.)

George House Trust is a voluntary HIV organization for the North-West which provides specific voluntary services to people with HIV in their own homes. George House Trust provides a number of services for women with HIV disease, including befriending, babysitting, shopping and transport. There is a weekly women-only session, and a new Lesbian Health Project has been launched.

The International Community of Women Living with HIV/AIDS
P.O. Box 2338
London W8 4ZG
Tel: 081 221 1316
Fax: 081 243 8481

This worldwide organization grew out of women's informal networking at international conferences on AIDS. It exists to overcome the isolation felt by many women with HIV, to exchange information, to encourage self-empowerment, and to ensure that women have a say in decisions which affect them, including policy, research and service provision.

Positively Women
5 Sebastian Street
London EC1V 0HE
Tel: 071 490 5515 (client services)
    071 490 2327 (helpline 12 noon to 2 p.m.)
    071 490 5501 (administration)
Fax: 071 490 1690

Positively Women offers support services run by women with HIV/AIDS for women with HIV/AIDS. Services provided include one-to-one counselling, support groups, hospital or home visits, and information on a wide range of issues.

Project for Advice, Counselling and Education (PACE)
34 Hartham Road
London N7
Tel: 071 251 2689

PACE is a non-profit organization of lesbians and gay men which provides professional counselling, psychotherapy, education, training and HIV prevention services.

Women and Medical Practice (WAMP)
40 Turnpike Lane
London N8 0PS
Tel: 081 365 8285
    081 888 2782 (administration)

WAMP is a health information and advice and counselling service managed by women representing a variety of backgrounds, cultures and experiences. Services provided include: pre- and post-HIV-test counselling, worried-well support sessions, a multi-ethnic befriending service, a drop-in vegetarian cafe, some holistic therapies, and pregnancy testing.

Women's HIV/AIDS Network
c/o Terrence Higgins Trust
52 Grays Inn Road
London WC1X 8JU

Women's HIV/AIDS Network is a forum for discussion for women working in the field.

Women's HIV/AIDS Network Scotland
64a Broughton Street
Edinburgh EH1 3SA
Tel: 031 557 5199

Women's HIV/AIDS Network Scotland organizes seminars and discussions, and produces a newsletter.

Notes on Contributors

Judy Bury has worked as a general practitioner, family planning doctor, sexual counsellor and HIV counsellor. She now works in a drugs project in Edinburgh and also teaches general practitioners about HIV/AIDS and about working with drug users. She has written extensively about medical aspects of women's health and is the author of *Teenage Pregnancy in Scotland* (Birth Control Trust 1984). As a member of the Scottish Women and HIV/AIDS Network she contributed to and jointly edited *Working with Women and AIDS* published by Routledge in 1992.

Kate Butcher came to health work in a very roundabout way; from a German and Spanish degree to teaching English as a second language. This took her to Southern India and Nepal, where for two years she taught English and German and volunteered in local clinics. She completed her Masters in Health Education and Promotion at Leeds, and has worked in health promotion for seven years, including working for three projects for women who work in prostitution. She helped set up the Bradford Working Women's Project, which now provides support, information, free condoms and needles and an advocacy service from its own premises in Bradford.

Sally Dowling trained as a psychiatric nurse and currently works as a Health Adviser in Bristol Royal Infirmary's Department of Genito-Urinary Medicine, offering counselling and advice on all sexual health matters including HIV/AIDS. She has an MA in Women's Studies, and has a longstanding interest in the emotional aspects of HIV infection for women. This is her first published work.

Lesley Doyal is Professor of Health Studies at the University of the West of England, Bristol. She has published extensively on health and health care and has a particular interest in gender and wellbeing. Her next book, *What Makes Women Sick? Gender and the Politics of Health* will be published by Macmillan in 1994.

Sheila Henderson is a freelance researcher and consultant with a particular interest in gender, health and lifestyle issues. She is currently working on a two-year project on Young Women's Recreational Drug Use and associated sexual and more general lifestyles in association with the Manchester drug agency Lifeline. She is an Honorary Research Fellow at Manchester University and has lectured on gender perspectives in history, sociology and cultural studies. Her publications are largely in the area of drug use, gender and HIV/AIDS.

Janet Holland is Senior Research Officer at the Department of Policy Studies, Institute of Education, University of London, with general interests in youth, gender and class. She is currently researching young men's sexuality (the Men, Risk and AIDS Project, MRAP) and evaluation of street drug agencies. She and her co-authors worked together as members of the Women, Risk and AIDS Project (WRAP).

Jenny Kitzinger is a lesbian feminist living in Scotland. She is currently working on The Child Abuse and the Media Project at Glasgow University Media Group (address for correspondence, 61 Southpark Avenue, Glasgow G12 8LF).

Michelle McCarthy has worked with people with learning difficulties for many years. She has also been involved with a number of feminist organizations and worked for five years on a Rape Crisis Line. For four years she specialized in working with women with learning difficulties on a sexuality project. She has greatly appreciated the opportunities this has given her to work with women with learning difficulties from a feminist perspective and to write about that work. She is now Lecturer in Learning Disability at the University of Kent at Canterbury.

Jennie Naidoo is a Senior Lecturer and Course Leader in Health Promotion at the University of the West of England, where she also teaches social sciences and Women's Studies. She has worked as a research officer and health promotion officer and is currently co-writing an introductory textbook on health promotion (Bailliere Tindall, forthcoming). Her research interests include women's health and health promotion, and she has published several articles in these areas.

Caroline Ramazanoglu is a senior lecturer in sociology at Goldsmith's College, University of London with interests in gender, race, power and methodology. Together with her co-authors, she is currently contributing to MRAP, and worked with them on the Women, Risk and AIDS Project.

Diane Richardson is Senior Lecturer in the Department of Sociological Studies at the University of Sheffield. She is the author of *Women and the AIDS Crisis* (Pandora Press, 1987, 2nd edition 1989) and *Safer Sex: The Guide for Women Today* (Pandora Press, 1990). Her other books include *The Theory and Practice of Homosexuality* (Routledge and Kegan Paul, 1981). *Women, Motherhood and Childrearing* (Macmillan, 1993) and, as co-editor, *Introducing Women's Studies: Feminist Theory and Practice* (Macmillan, 1993). She has also written plays and short stories.

Sue Scott is senior lecturer in sociology at the University of Stirling. Her main research interests are feminist methodology, the application of sociology to evaluation and the sociology of mind, body and emotion. Together with her co-authors she contributed to the Women, Risk and AIDS Project.

Sue Sharpe is a freelance writer, researcher and consultant, whose main interests are the lives and experiences of young women including work on young men and heterosexuality. Her books include *Just Like a Girl* (Penguin, 1976), *Falling for Love* (Virago, 1987) and *Voices from Home* (Virago, 1990). Together with her co-authors, she is currently contributing to MRAP.

Rachel Thomson is Senior Development Officer for the Sex Education Forum at the National Children's Bureau. Together with her co-authors she worked on the Women, Risk and AIDS Project and is currently contributing to MRAP.

Tamsin Wilton is Senior Lecturer in Health Studies at the University of the West of England, where she also teaches Women's Studies. She has been involved in HIV/AIDS and safer sex training both in a voluntary and professional capacity since 1987. She is the author of *Antibody Politic — AIDS and Society* (New Clarion Press, 1992) and of *A Lesbian Studies Primer* (Routledge, forthcoming), the co-author of *AIDS — Working with Young People* (AVERT, 1990/1993) and has written widely on HIV/AIDS and on sexuality. She is currently editing a book on lesbians and cinema for Routledge, and writing *Engendering AIDS: The Sexual Politics of an Epidemic,* to be published by Falmer Press.

Index

abortion 23, 33, 54, 62, 71, 167
ACT UP 47, 55
adolescence 85, 122–45
advertising for AIDS campaign 51, 103–7
Advisory Council on Misuse of Drugs 185, 187
Africa 1, 12–13, 102
  economic dependence of women 11–17
  prevention programmes 18–19, 25
  prostitution 15, 25, 152
AIDS Counselling and Education (ACE) 25
AIDS-Related Complex (ARC) 36
alcohol 156, 184, 185, 191–2
American Moral Majority 90
amphetamines 186, 192
anal intercourse 31, 86, 160, 163
  learning difficulties 173–4, 178–80
anorexia nervosa 72
antidepressants 184
appearance of young women 68–71, 76
Asia 12, 17, 25
  prostitution 16, 25, 152
Australia 1, 46, 88
AZT (Zidovudine) 39, 183

babies 20
  drug trials 21–2
  drug use in pregnancy 184, 189
  transmission of HIV from mother 5, 22, 30–5, 45, 102, 115–16, 167
bastard syndrome 133–7, 140
bisexual men 36, 83, 96, 98–9, 103, 168
bisexual women 53, 161, 162
blood transfusions
  lesbians refused as donors 114, 159
  transmission of HIV 30–2, 34, 36, 102, 117, 162

Brazil 23
breast cancer 47, 48
breast-feeding 33, 34–5
Brooklyn AIDS Task Force (BATF) 25

CAL-PEP project 154
Cameroon 25
cancer 36, 38
  breast 47, 48
  cervical 37, 39, 47, 52, 87
candida 36
candidiasis 36
cannabis 192
carers, women 3, 6–7, 24, 42, 45, 54, 99
  mental health 113, 115, 116, 118
celibacy 72
Centers for Disease Control (CDC) 37, 161–2
Central Funding Initiative (CFI) 186, 187
cervical cancer 37, 39, 47, 52, 87
cervical cell abnormalities 23, 37
cervical dysplasia 37
chancroid 13, 21
childbearing 30, 32–5, 115–16
  see also reproductive activities
childcare 50, 54, 113, 118
  lesbians 167
  women drug users 185
children 15, 20, 34, 42, 115, 118
  infected by mothers 22, 102
  of lesbians 165
  number infected 12
  see also babies
chlamydia 21, 163
class, social 4, 14, 95, 99, 101–2
  drug use 192
  lesbians 169

masculinity 123, 125, 144
prostitution 156
clitoris 66, 86, 174
colour 4, 17, 21, 31
AIDS discourse 95, 99, 101–3, 105, 107
lesbians 166
masculinity 123, 144
prevention programmes 18–19, 25
prostitution 15, 156
survival 23, 38
see also ethnicity; race
Community Drug Teams (CDTs) 188
condoms 32, 51–2, 83
AIDS discourse 96, 105–6
drug users 188
female 25
femininity 70–1
learning difficulties 173, 176, 180
lesbians 164, 166
prevention programmes 18–20, 25
prostitution 154, 155
contraception 1, 48, 53, 62, 66, 70
counselling services 116–19
drugs 188, 190
Coyote 155
cunnilingus 86, 161, 164, 179

dance drugs 192–3
ddI (new drug on trial) 39
dental dams 86, 164, 173
diagnosis of HIV/AIDS
babies and children 34
women 23, 35–8, 43, 49, 113, 115–16, 119
Diana, Princess 80, 99
discrimination towards lesbians 165, 168
domination of women 89, 140–1
see also oppression of women; power relations; subordination of women
Dominican Republic 25
double standards 140–3, 168
dramas about AIDS 100–1
Drug Dependency Units (DDUs) 188
Drug Misuse Databases 187
drug trials 21–2, 37, 39, 113, 167
drugs, illicit 7, 17–18, 178
AIDS discourse 95–7, 102, 106
lesbians 160–3, 165, 168
prostitution 156, 184, 188
survival 23, 38
transmission of HIV 12, 30–2, 36, 162
use by women 35, 45, 183–93
Drugs, Alcohol, Women, Nationally (DAWN) 185, 188

economic dependence of women 14–17, 18
Ecstasy 192
education *see* health education; sex education
effeminacy 128, 132
Empower Project 26, 155
empowerment of women 65, 75
prostitution 152, 155
English Collective of Prostitutes 155
eroticism and health promotion 80–91
ethnicity 20–1, 123, 125, 192
see also colour; race
Europe 1–2, 11, 12, 44

faeces 31
fellatio 86, 179
femininity 6, 68–72, 75, 76, 125, 144
health promotion 89–90
fidelity and faithfulness 14, 19
finger-fucking 86
first sexual encounters of young men 124, 126, 129, 131, 133–5, 144
older women 126, 137–9
Foucault, M. 62–5, 75, 84, 88–90
funding 2–3
drug programmes 186, 187, 188
gay support services 167, 169
research 22, 38

gay men 1, 7, 46–8, 123, 144, 166–9
AIDS counselling 116–18
AIDS discourse 95–6, 98–101, 103, 106
criticism of lesbians 159
health care 22, 30, 36, 83–6, 89–91, 168–9
homophobia 114
support groups 1–2, 166–7, 169
transmission of HIV 12, 30–1
see also homosexuals
gender 3–4, 8
drugs use 185–7, 193
health care 20–1, 26
inequalities 14–15, 24
power relations 62–5, 75, 82, 127, 152–3, 176
prevention programmes 18–20
progression of AIDS 22, 38
genital herpes 12, 37
genital ulceration 13, 31
genital warts 31, 37
gladiators 122, 131–3, 135, 143–4
sexual reputation 140, 143
gonorrhoea 13, 21, 31, 103
gynaecological infections 21, 37
drug trials 39

health care 45, 54, 100
  gay men 22, 30, 36, 83–6, 89–91, 168–9
  lesbians 159, 160, 169
  promotion 80–91, 151
  survival 38
  women with AIDS 20–6
  see also women's health movement
health education 1–3, 5, 75, 164, 168–9
  AIDS policies 47–51
  learning difficulties 173, 176
  lesbians 159, 163, 166
  media advertisements 103–7
  prevention of HIV transmission 24–6
  prostitution 151, 152, 154–5
  women 45, 50, 54
Health Education Authority 51, 80, 107
heroin 183, 184, 186, 190
herpes 12, 23, 37, 163
heterosexual intercourse
  challenging sexual risk 75–6
  double standards 168
  drugs 17–18
  economic dependence of women 14–17
  female sexuality 72–5
  femininity 68–71
  gender inequalities 14, 24
  health promotion 86–9
  learning difficulties 173–6, 178–81
  lesbians 160–3
  masculinity of young men 122–45
  negotiations 5, 14, 45, 62, 65, 75, 80, 90
  pleasure 87–8
  poverty 17–18
  power relations 3–6, 50–1, 53–5, 62–5,
    75–6
  prevention programmes 18–20
  prostitution 155, 157
  safer sex 51, 61
  sexual education 65–7
  transmission of HIV 2, 5, 12–13, 30–2,
    51–2, 114, 116
homophobia 81, 83–4, 88, 91, 114
homosexuals 2
  AIDS discourse 95–6, 98, 100, 106
  health promotion 80, 85, 86
  learning difficulties 174
  masculinity of young men 128
  see also gay men; lesbians
housing 49, 54, 118
  lesbians 165, 167
  women drug users 188–90
Human Fertilisation and Embryology Act
  (1990) 165

image
  young men 126–7, 130–2
  young women 68–71, 76
India 16, 25, 153
insemination 32, 160, 165–6
International Community of Women
    Living with HIV/AIDS 1–2
International Congress for Prostitutes'
    Rights 153, 156

Kaposi's sarcoma (KS) 36, 38
Kenya 25, 152
kerbcrawling 153
kissing 31

learning difficulties 7, 171–81
lesbians 44–5, 53–4, 159–69, 191
  AIDS discourse 95–6, 98, 101, 106
  AIDS politics 46–7
  health promotion 84, 86, 89, 90
  mental health 114–15, 118
  prostitution 156
  sadomasochism 55, 164
  safer sex 44, 96, 160, 164, 166
  transmission of HIV 5, 7, 30, 31, 44,
    160–4, 168
Lesbian AIDS Project 161
lesions 113
literature
  lesbians 159–61, 167
  mental health 119
  women with AIDS 43–5
  women and drugs 184
Local Government Act (1988)(section 28)
  165
LSD 192

masculinity 6, 75
  bastard syndrome 133–7, 140
  double standards 140–3
  older women 126, 137–40
  peer groups 126, 128–33, 138, 143
  power 125–6, 143–4
  sexual identity 83, 86, 90
  young men 122–45
masturbation 66–7, 80, 174
media
  advertisements 103–7
  homophobia 114
  lesbians 46, 159, 166
  prostitution 151
  women and AIDS 95–6, 99–107
  women and drugs 183–4
Men, Risk and AIDS Project (MRAP) 124,
  125

menstruation 23, 69, 73, 140, 163
  drug trials 39
  HIV in blood 32, 163
mental health 6, 113–19
methadone 183, 186
Mexico 25
mothers 3–6, 20, 22–3
  AIDS discourse 95–102, 106
  of infected children 117–18
  infecting children 22, 102
  transmission to babies 5, 22, 30–5, 45,
    102, 115–16, 167

needles and syringes
  exchanges 186, 187, 188
  sharing 30, 32, 36, 161, 163
negotiations in sex 5, 14, 45, 62, 65, 75, 80,
  90
  learning difficulties 173, 176, 178, 180
  lesbians 164
  safer sex 14, 51
  young men 124–5, 143–4
Nigeria 25
non-penetrative sex 20, 52, 106, 179
  health promotion 83, 90
numbers of HIV infected people 2, 11–12,
  12

Oceania 17
older women 126, 137–40
opportunistic infections 36
oppression of women 5, 8, 45, 53, 62, 75,
  114
  health promotion 81–2, 84
  see also domination of women; power
    relations; subordination of women
oral sex 31–2, 86, 161, 164, 173, 179
orgasms, female 66, 73–4, 174
OutRage 47

patriarchy 13–14, 63, 64, 75
  health promotion 83, 84, 90
peer groups of young men 126, 128–33,
  138, 143
pelvic infection 21, 37, 39
penetrative sex 50, 179
  health promotion 86, 88, 90
  young men 126–7, 134
  see also heterosexual intercourse
People First 177
performance stories 128–33, 135
Philippines 154
Pneumocystis carinii pneumonia (PCP) 21,
  36, 114

pornography 5, 52–3, 55, 81–3, 86, 88–91
  safer sex 52, 53, 90–1
Positively Women 1, 119
poverty 17–18, 20, 38
power relations 45, 70, 73, 80
  gender 62–5, 75, 82, 127, 152–3, 176
  health promotion 84–5, 89, 90–1
  heterosexual 3–6, 50–1, 53–5, 62–5, 75–6
  older women 139
  pornography 82, 86
  young men 122–7, 130, 133, 137, 143–4
pregnancy 42, 45, 48, 51, 53, 54, 126
  diagnosis of AIDS 23
  drug trials 21–2, 39
  drugs use 183, 184, 188–9
  ectopic 21
  femininity 70–1
  health promotion 87
  HIV positive women 22, 33, 35, 102,
    116, 118
  learning difficulties 172
  lesbians 163
  medical issues 32–5
  progression of AIDS 22, 33, 35
  prostitution 156
  sex education 66
  STDs 21
  see also babies
prevention programmes 18–20, 24–6, 43,
  52–3, 177, 193
  prostitution 25–6, 151–2
progression of AIDS
  gender 22, 38
  pregnancy 22, 33, 35
promiscuity 95, 102, 116, 168
prostitution 2, 4, 6–7, 45, 151–7
  Africa 15, 25, 152
  AIDS discourse 95–6, 102–3, 104
  Asia 16, 25, 152
  double standards 168
  drugs 156, 184, 188
  prevention programmes 25–6, 151–2
  transmission of HIV 25, 31–2, 42, 53,
    151–2, 155

Queer Nation 47

race 3–4, 14, 45, 106–7
  drug use 192
  health care 21
  lesbians 169
  see also colour; ethnicity
rape 15, 16, 53, 54, 72, 87, 163
  condom use 154

reproductive activities 3, 49, 63, 67
    lesbians 165-7
    rights 45, 49, 54, 167
    see also childbearing
research 22, 38
Rwanda 19, 21

sadomasochism (lesbian) 55, 164
safer sex 5-7, 61-2
    AIDS discourse 105, 106
    feminist issues 45, 48, 52-4
    health promotion 81-91
    knowledge 68, 76
    learning difficulties 171-81
    lesbians 44, 96, 160, 164, 166
    negotiations 14, 51
    pornography 52, 53, 90-1
    power relations 62, 64-5
    prevention programmes 18-19
    prostitution 155
    sexual pleasure 87-8
    violence 54
    young men 144
saliva 31
semen 13, 31
seroconversion 31, 34-5
sex education 64, 65-7, 76
    learning difficulties 171-2, 175-81
    young men 126-7
sex toys 164
sex workers 2, 15, 151
    prevention programmes 25-6
    see also prostitution
sexual abuse 16, 48, 53, 72, 87
    learning difficulties 7, 172, 174-6
    lesbians 163
sexual identity 83-7, 90, 123
sexual reputation 126, 140-3
sexually transmitted diseases (STDs) 21,
    26, 66, 70
    clinics 119
    feminists 51, 52-3
    learning difficulties 172
    lesbians 163
    poverty 17
    transmission of HIV 13, 31
    young men 124
slimming pills 184, 186
Society for Women and AIDS 1
sterilization 54, 102
subordination of women 6, 65, 74-6, 82, 91
    prostitution 152
    young men 125-6, 144
    see also domination of women;

oppression of women; power relations
support organizations 1-2, 113-14, 166-7,
    169
survival of women with AIDS 20-1, 23, 38
symptoms of HIV/AIDS
    gender differences 22
    in pregnancy 33
    women 5, 33, 35-7, 114
syphilis 13, 21, 51, 103

Terrence Higgins Trust 43-4, 85, 118, 164
Thailand 16, 25, 26, 154, 155
thrush 23, 36-7, 39, 163
tobacco and smoking 184, 191-2
tranquillizers 184, 186
transmission of HIV 99, 100-2
    blood transfusion 30-2, 34, 36, 102, 117,
    162
    drug use 12, 30-2, 36, 162
    feminist issues 42, 44-5, 51-3
    gay men 12, 30-1
    health promotion 80-1, 86
    heterosexual 2, 5, 12-13, 30-2, 51-2, 114,
    116
    learning difficulties 173, 178
    lesbian sex 5, 7, 30, 31, 44, 160-4, 168
    mother to baby 5, 22, 30-5, 45, 102, 115-
    16, 167
    oral sex 30, 31, 173
    prevention 18-20, 24-6, 43, 52-3, 151-2,
    177, 193
    promiscuity 116
    prostitution 25, 31-2, 42, 53, 151-2, 155
    sharing needles 30, 32, 36
    STDs 13, 31
    by women 42, 96

Uganda 16, 19-21, 152
United States 1-2, 12, 17, 90
    benefits for AIDS sufferers 37
    health care 20-3
    learning difficulties 171, 174
    lesbians 44, 161-2, 165
    prevention programmmes 18-19, 25
    prostitution 155
    survival 38
Urban Health Study 161
urine 31

vaginal secretions 13, 31, 32, 163
venereal disease 103, 151
videos for education 173, 180
violence 16, 18, 54, 63, 72, 76
    learning difficulties 179

lesbians 164
prostitution 156
virginity 124, 126, 129, 131, 133–5, 137–9

wimps 122, 128, 132–3, 135, 143–4
Women, Risk and AIDS Project (WRAP)
   65
   sexual reputation 140, 142
   young men's masculinity 124–6, 139

women's health movement 2–4, 47–8, 50
   illicit drugs 183, 184–6
   lesbians 169
World Whores' Congress 156

Zaire 18, 116
Zambia 21
Zimbabwe 17, 21, 152

Printed in the United Kingdom
by Lightning Source UK Ltd.
106524UKS00002BA/6

9 780748 401635